1987

The Corporatization of Health Care Delivery

The Hospital-Physician Relationship

Compiled by

Monica R. Dreuth
American Hospital Association
Division of Medical Affairs

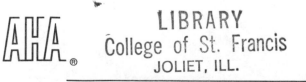

American Hospital Publishing, Inc.,
a wholly owned subsidiary of the
American Hospital Association

Library of Congress Cataloging in Publication Data

The Corporatization of health care delivery.
  "Catalog no. 145136"—T.p. verso.
  An outgrowth of a conference sponsored by
the American Hospital Association and its
Council on Hospital Medical Staffs, held July
27-28, 1985.
    1. Hospitals—Medical staff—Congresses.
2.Hospital-physician joint ventures—
Congresses.   3. Medical corporations—
Congresses.   4. Hospitals—Sociological
aspects—Congresses.   I. Dreuth, Monica R.
II. American Hospital Association.   III. Council
on Hospital Medical Staffs (American Hospital
Association)   [DNLM: 1.   Hospital Administration
—congresses.   2.   Interprofessional Relations—
congresses.   3.   Medical Staff, Hospital—
organization & administration.   WX 160 C822]
RA972.C67   1986   362.1'1'0683   86-14124

ISBN 0-939450-94-1

Catalog no. 145136

©1986 by American Hospital Publishing, Inc.
a wholly owned subsidiary
of the American Hospital Association

AHA is a service mark of American Hospital Association used under license by
American Hospital Publishing, Inc.

Printed in the U.S.A.
2.5M-8/86-0144

Audrey Kaufman, Editor
Peggy DuMais, Production Coordinator
Brian Schenk, Acquisitions and Editorial Manager
Dorothy Saxner, Vice-President, Books

Contents

List of Figures

Foreword

The central theme that emerges from these pages is that physicians must actively participate in the future of health care delivery. The critical dimension of quality control is the most natural, appropriate, and pivotal locus for physician involvement. Those who ignore involvement at this level do so at their peril.

Physicians as patient advocates must learn and teach rigorous methods of quality assessment and assurance and must be able to demonstrate to intelligent lay persons the importance that these qualitative and quantitative data reflect. A failure of physicians to carry out this task has the potential not only to cause the failure of corporate medicine but to cause the failure of the profession of medicine itself.

The Corporatization of Health Care Delivery examines hospital-physician relationships against the backdrop of the current growth of health care systems. Shortell begins with his analysis of an environment in which physicians and hospitals are simultaneously being pushed together and pulled apart, giving rise to relationships that are characterized by paradox, ambiguity and change, and risk. He proposes three new medical staff organizational models for the future and discusses the assets and liabilities of each.

Egdahl and Taft observe that one difference between the past and the present is a much greater sharing of financial risk by physicians and hospitals. They are convinced that the hospital's central mission will continue to be its inpatient services, but that more care will be provided in the ambulatory setting. They predict that underutilization of health services will soon be a major issue, and they urge that procedures be developed to identify it.

Landgarten's discussion of joint ventures highlights a variety of potential risks and benefits for hospitals and physicians. Both he and Lewis discuss ways to create a climate that is receptive to change. Lewis cautions against using joint ventures as a ''quick fix'' to resolve hospital-physician relationship problems, and he shares some commonsense advice on open dialogue and mutual trust.

In the chapter by Roeder and Moxley, the reader is taken on a historical journey from the acute care hospital of the 19th Century to today's vertically integrated health care system. They point to the medical staff's clinical expertise and responsibility for assuring quality of care as crucial noneconomic elements in the health care system.

Jencks then discusses federal trends for physician payment. Perhaps the best news is his conclusion that because there have been dramatic changes in some areas of the country and no changes in other areas, federal approaches must remain flexible lest they produce more harm than good. Although this chapter was written before Congress renewed its interest in examining different physician payment mechanisms, it is worthy of review, as some of the data run counter to present perceptions of reality.

The concluding two chapters explore legal issues of growing concern to hospitals and their medical staffs. Hughes reviews judicial findings on institutional responsibility for physician practices within the hospital, and Jessee focuses on prescriptions to limit, or at least decrease, exposure to malpractice liability. Their advice to have diligent, responsive department chairmen and solid review mechanisms for quality of care and credentialing is particularly important in the current climate of escalating malpractice suits.

One suspects that the current headlong rush to corporatization may too often be a rush to simple commercialization. The chapter that remains to be written in real life is on the reality of caring for human needs within a commercial paradigm. This is a challenge that administrators, trustees, and physicians must face together. *The Corporatization of Health Care Delivery* identifies some of the crucial issues facing hospital administration and medical staffs today and provides practical suggestions for their working together to meet this challenge.

Don E. Detmer, M.D.
Vice-President for Health Services
University of Utah

Preface

The Corporatization of Health Care Delivery is an outgrowth of an annual conference on medical staff issues, sponsored by the American Hospital Association and its Council on Hospital Medical Staffs. The conference is part of a continuing effort to encourage dialogue between administrators, trustees, and medical staff leaders on trends and issues that have an impact on hospital-physician relationships.

We hope that the ideas set forth in these pages will serve as a starting point for thoughtful discussion. Although there is no panacea or "quick fix" in this complex environment, where physicians and hospitals are both competitors and partners, it is hoped that this book will provide some guidance on how to meld financial concerns with concerns for quality of care. In addition, a variety of models are proposed that would reshape the traditional medical staff organization, making way for joint ventures, shared risk taking, and increased opportunities for physicians to participate in institutional governance.

We wish to express our appreciation to the individuals whose work appears on the following pages and to the members of the Council on Hospital Medical Staffs for their support of the American Hospital Association's efforts to foster collaborative relationships between hospitals and physicians. We hope that this book will make a contribution to that objective and that it will be used as a catalyst for local decision making at leadership retreats, board meetings, and medical staff meetings.

Monica R. Dreuth
Director
AHA Division of Medical Affairs

Chapter 1

New Models for Hospital-Physician Relations

Stephen M. Shortell, Ph.D.

The ability of hospitals and physicians to forge effective new relationships will shape the delivery of health services over the remainder of the century. The current relationship, based on the voluntary medical staff organization structure, is largely unable to deal with the changing health care environment.

The Underlying Issues

Cost containment pressures, increased competition, the "corporatization" of health care, and the growth of health care teams are at one and the same time pushing hospitals and physicians closer together and yet farther apart. They give rise to characteristics of paradox, ambiguity and change, risk, and "responsible excellence."

Paradox

The relationships between hospitals and physicians are increasingly *paradoxical* (and will become more so) in that they are *both* competitors and collaborators. It is inherently a love-hate relationship. Many hospitals are directly competing with physicians to maintain or expand market share through developing ambulatory care centers, emergicenters, sports medicine clinics, health promotion programs, and related initiatives. At the same time, physicians are developing similar activities in order to maintain their patient base. Although competition takes place in these areas, collaboration exists in other areas where both physicians and hospitals see mutual advantages (that is, where both can maintain or increase market share or competitive advantage). Examples include some HMO developments, some preferred provider organization arrangements, independent practice associations, and similar joint ventures.

Dr. Shortell is Professor of Hospital and Health Services Management, Northwestern University, Evanston, IL.

Reprinted, with permission, from *CHA Insight.* 1985 Feb. 9(5):1-6. A portion of this chapter was also reprinted, with permission, from *Frontiers of Health Services Management.* 1985 Feb. 1(3):3-48.

In some cases, hospitals compete with particular subsets of their medical staff while collaborating with others. In other cases, the *same people* are involved as both competitors and collaborators: particularly in multihospital communities. The relevant question for managers and physicians is not "How do we avoid competing with each other?" but, rather, "On what basis will the competition take place?" To what degree will both parties be able to deal with it in a constructive fashion? The relevant question, thus, becomes: "When and where does it make sense for us to compete and when and where is it best for us to collaborate?"

Managers and physicians need to become more comfortable about agreeing to disagree without losing respect and trust. They also need to recognize the difference between short-run competition and long-run collaboration. For example, current pressures may dictate some degree of competition between hospitals and physicians in the short-run but the long-run interdependencies between hospitals and physicians suggest the need for collaboration. In fact, it is not only possible but likely that out of competition will come collaboration. This is because when two parties compete with each other, they learn more about each other's comparative advantage, which, in turn, leads to possibilities of joint undertakings; particularly as additional "third parties" enter the market. Thus, one observes some hospitals and physicians jointly operating renal dialysis centers, home health agencies, ambulatory surgicenters, and emergicenters in areas where they formerly competed as individual entities. This occurs where each party perceives that a comparative advantage can be gained through a joint undertaking.

Another dimension of the paradox is to recognize that the hospital medical staff organization structure has dual socialization responsibilities; it is *both* a socializing unit for the *profession and practice of medicine* and a socializing unit for the *hospital as an organization*. In recent years, the latter function has become increasingly important. The question of whether the current traditional medical staff organization structure is capable of doing this or whether new models are needed is discussed in a later section. It is of significance to note that research on professionals in other industries suggests that the most highly motivated are those who are *both* "local" (that is, having a high commitment to the organization) and "cosmopolitan" (that is, having a high commitment to the profession).[1, 2] What has been true for many scientists in industry is now true for physicians in hospitals. One of the keys to success will be the ability to fulfill this dual socialization responsibility.

Ambiguity and Change

The relationship between hospitals and physicians is also becoming increasingly *ambiguous* and filled with *change*. For example, the nature of the mutual dependencies is changing. In some ways hospitals are becoming more dependent on physicians not only to fill beds with the right kinds of patients

but to deal with risk management and complex clinical/bioethical/adminis-
trative issues, such as Baby Doe cases. In other ways, such as staff admitting
privileges, hospitals are becoming less dependent because of the growing
surplus of physicians. Hospitals can be more choosy about who they admit
to the staff, and they can demand more of those to whom they grant
privileges.

   Similar dependencies exist for physicians. They are becoming more
dependent on hospitals as competition for privileges increases. The specialists,
in particular, require access to the expensive technology and support services that only hospitals can provide. In addition, trained primary care
physicians are also increasingly dependent on hospitals for assistance in
developing their practices (for example, through subsidized rent leases or
formal sponsorship, provision of billing, and support services). Yet in other
ways, physicians are less dependent on hospitals; particularly as less inva-
sive out-of-hospital technology (for example, home renal dialysis, fiber-
optics, ultrasound) is developed, which can be used in physician offices or in
the patient's home. Further, some physicians joining urgicenters,
emergicenters, and free-standing ambulatory surgery centers are only interested in providing acute general medical care and do not seek hospital
privileges. They have learned that there are other ways of capturing referral
markets. The ambiguity created by such conflicting dependencies between
hospitals and physicians affects every major hospital policy decision and
must be explicitly recognized by both parties.

   The age and specialty mix of the hospital staff gives rise to further
ambiguity, and complicates the change process. Physicians' views differ
depending on the issue involved. For example, specialists will typically
support (or at least not actively oppose) hospital efforts to develop additional
primary care programs that will channel more patient referrals to the
hospital specialists. Support for such programs, however, is likely to be in
direct relationship to the amount of opposition and leverage that can be
mustered by the existing primary care physicians on staff who currently
refer patients to the specialists. The ability of primary care physicians to
have such economic clout over a given hospital's specialty staff depends on
the number of primary care physicians involved, the value of their referrals,
their relative influence on the staff, the availability of other specialists in the
community (to whom they could switch their referrals), and the availability
of alternative sources of referrals for the specialists.

   In similar fashion, conflicts occur along age lines. Although somewhat
over-simplified, physician concerns regarding hospital behavior can be roughly
broken down into three age groups: recently trained physicians,
approximately 1 to 5 years out of their residencies; a middle group,
approximately 6 to 20 years out of their residencies; and an older group,
over 20 years away from their residency training. The older group, many
with long established practices and some looking toward retirement, are
generally least concerned and least affected by the current pressures. The

younger group (1 to 5 years out) are concerned and very much affected by the changes, but, in effect, have "grown up" with the changes. They also have different expectations for their professional careers than their older colleagues. More of them tend to prefer practicing in groups and many see competitive advantages to developing contractual relationships and other linkages with hospitals. They also tend to have somewhat more modest income expectations than their earlier trained colleagues and are more willing to trade off large incomes for more regular work hours, leisure time, and family life. A growing percentage of physicians are women (approximately 33 percent of all graduates in 1985), who are more favorably predisposed toward institution-based practice and more regular hours. It is among these younger men and women that the medical staff leadership of tomorrow will emerge. The wise manager will begin investing in them now.

The "in-between" group (roughly 6 to 20 years out) are the most upset and affected by the changes. They are also the least able to cope. They entered their professional careers with some of the same expectations as their older colleagues, but have, in effect, had the rug pulled out from under them before they have had a chance to achieve their objectives. It is from this group that most managers are experiencing conflict and unrest. The overall emotional climate of a given hospital's medical-staff relationship can largely be judged by the size of this in-between group. It is often exacerbated because it is from this group that the medical staff's formal leaders (chief of staff, clinical chiefs, committee chairs, and so forth) are most frequently found.

Thus, depending on the issue, these three different groups will frequently have conflicting views, lending additional ambiguity to the situation. Of course, many situations are even more complex in that the split does not take place along age lines alone but will cut across specialties as noted above and in other cases, informal colleague networks and sponsorship processes.[3-5]

Risk

Hospital-physician relationships are increasingly characterized by greater *risk*. Because the environment is more paradoxical and ambiguous, it is more difficult to guarantee the success of new initiatives or even attach a reasonable probability. Decisions are more "inspirational" in the sense of not understanding cause and effect relationships nor agreeing on what would constitute desirable outcomes. And because of cost containment and competitive pressures, the stakes are higher. For some institutions it is a matter of survival.

For three reasons, the issue of taking on more risk is particularly problematic for hospitals. First, it is novel. In the era of cost-based reimbursement, the relative lack of competition, and strong community philanthropic support, hospitals could launch new efforts without having to assume much risk.

Second, the very nature of clinical decision making that undergirds hospital behavior is inherently conservative. In order to avoid the type I error of not diagnosing someone who is ill, all efforts have traditionally been made to diagnose illness and to "take no chances." This clinical mentality of "taking no chances" and striving for perfection is carried over to administrative decision making in which administrators have been hesitant to take risks for fear that failure would be upsetting to the board, or medical staff, or both. Conservatism is inherent in most hospitals and is consistent with their medical missions.

Third, hospital trustees, many of whom are entrepreneurial-minded business men and women, mysteriously seem to lose their penchant for taking risks once they assume their seats on the hospital board. Their behavior suggests that they have had their fill of such activity in their own businesses and that their membership on the hospital board really represents their community service. They also dislike conflict. Many view the hospital as a voluntary, charitable institution in which entrepreneurship, risk taking, and tough management practices have little place. Until recently, this view was reinforced by the administrative and clinical mentality of administrators and physicians, as noted above. This mind-set is now out of tune with the times. A key ingredient in the development of more successful hospital-physician relationships in the future will be the ability of trustees, management, and physicians to embrace risk. The danger lies not in failure per se but in the failure to learn from new experiences. Successful relationships in the future will not only be based on trust but on the ability to maximize the learning that takes place from engaging in some degree of risky behavior.

Responsible Excellence—Comparative Advantage

Finally, paradox, ambiguity/change, and risk call for *responsible excellence*. Responsible excellence means learning what one does best and having the wisdom to leave to others what they do best. Or, put differently, learning to recognize and capitalize on one's comparative advantage. The idea is similar to Norton's idea of a *congeniality of excellences* wherein one learns to appreciate and enjoy the different gifts which each party possesses.[6] In the present environment of constrained resources it is no longer possible for individual hospitals to be "the best at everything." They must do a more rigorous job of environmental assessment, competitive analysis, organizational assessment, and market analysis to determine those areas of comparative advantage where the hospital and its medical staff should be striving for excellence. Most important, this needs to be done with relevant involvement of the medical staff. Assessment of the strengths and weaknesses and competitive advantages of one's staff is key to the development of effective relationships and the pursuit of responsible excellence.

Comparative advantage, or responsible excellence, also includes the notion of community welfare. What is best for the hospital may not be best for the community. Constructive competition between hospitals and physicians may provide worthwhile options for the community. For example, some emergicenters have been successful because they have met the community's desire for more accessible and convenient care. The notion of community responsibility also means that hospitals need to know when to compete and when to collaborate with other hospitals and health care organizations. One's own physicians and the physicians associated with other organizations (some, of course, may be one and the same) are central to the unfolding of these strategic decisions.

New Models for Hospital-Physician Relations

The implication of paradox, ambiguity and change, risk, and comparative advantage is that they are not to be avoided but, rather, embraced. They must be explicitly designed into new medical staff organizational structures and in new partnerships between hospitals and physicians. Prospective payment, competition, technological growth, and changing public expectations call for new mechanisms for dealing with these underlying issues and for fostering professional and organizational learning. Three new models for consideration are the independent-corporate model, the divisional model, and the parallel model.

Independent-Corporate Model

In this model, the medical staff is a separate legal entity that negotiates with the hospital for the provision of services. There are no *hospital* medical staff bylaws, credentialing, quality assurance or related mechanisms. These functions are conducted exclusively by the independent group of physicians that contracts with the hospital (figure 1.1, next page). In a competitive market, the physician group may develop quality assurance and cost containment features to contract with the more desirable hospitals in the community. These might well go beyond current standards set by the Joint Commission on Accreditation of Hospitals and other licensing and regulatory bodies.

A variation of the independent-corporate model—prepaid health care in the *group model* health maintenance organization (HMO)—has a long history. The classic example is the Kaiser Permanente Medical Group, which contracts with the Kaiser Health Plan. Many hospitals are moving towards this kind of relationship with their medical staffs in developing preferred provider organizations (PPOs) and related joint ventures. However, these arrangements are usually overlaid on the traditional medical staff structure. The independent-corporate model involves complete legal separation of hospital and physicians.

Figure 1.1. The Independent-Corporate Model

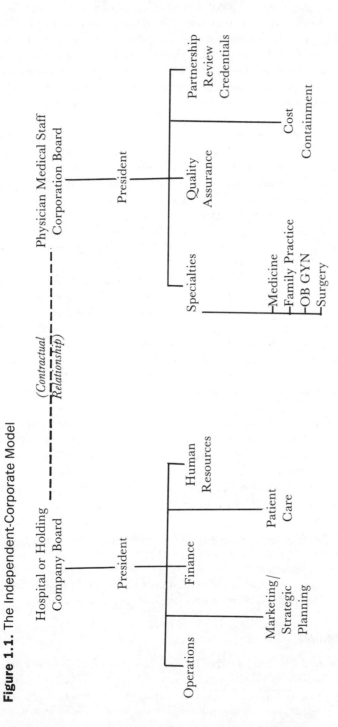

Where existing hospital-physician medical staff relationships have deteriorated, a legal separation may be a "fresh start" for both parties. For the hospital, it may permit more efficient organization of patient care and administrative support functions. The power, authority, influence, and perhaps effectiveness of the nursing staff may increase. In communities with several large multispecialty group practices, such a separation may allow negotiations with the different groups for favorable cost and quality arrangements.

However, a separation is extremely risky because the hospital loses control over the medical staff. It may be more difficult to coordinate the nursing, ancillary service, and physician care components of patient treatment. Monitoring arm's length relationships with medical corporations also requires considerable time and effort.

The main advantage to physicians is increased autonomy. An independent legal entity gives physicians sole responsibility for developing their own governing bylaws, quality assurance, and credentialing mechanisms. Physicians could also monitor members' use, cost, and quality of care performance. Further, physicians would be out from under the accreditation, licensing, and regulatory apparatus directed at hospitals. (Nothing, of course, prevents these groups from turning their attention to the independent medical staff corporations.) Many physicians might also prefer dealing with these third parties directly rather than be represented by the hospital.

One disadvantage is that hospital-based physicians may not be able to purchase malpractice insurance at the rates they received through the hospital. Older physicians with established loyalty to the hospital may also perceive disadvantages. Younger physicians, women physicians, physicians of minority ethnic backgrounds, and foreign-trained physicians might lose protections afforded by the checks and balances of a formal hospital medical staff structure. Power may be unduly concentrated in the clinical chiefs of independent medical corporations.

The complete legal separation of hospital and medical staff might increase each group's ability to respond quickly to issues that primarily affect only one party—but each would be handicapped on issues requiring collaboration. Further, there are considerable differences among physicians over specialty training, experience, and practice styles, all of which make it difficult for entirely separate corporations to develop. Thus, the pure independent-corporate model is unlikely to be a viable alternative in many communities. Nonetheless, it represents one end of the continuum.

Divisional Model

The divisional model is characterized by the placement of such functions as finance, nursing, personnel, and marketing within each division, organized in figure 1.2 (next page) along clinical specialty lines. Divisions could also be organized around groups of several specialties, such as a primary care

Figure 1.2. The Divisional Model (Traditional Specialties)

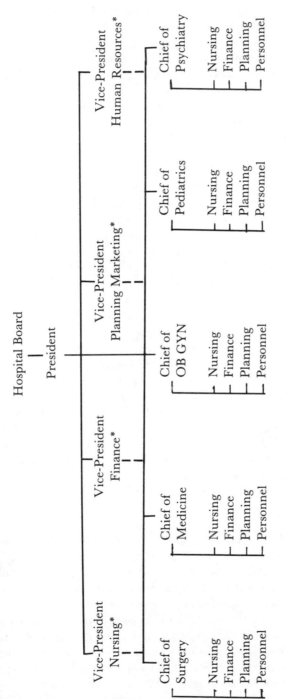

*Vice Presidents report to the President, advise division Chiefs.

division, an acute medical/surgical division, a chronic care division, and a specialized services division, or around specific product/service lines, such as musculoskeletal, gastrointestinal, cardiovascular, nervous system, and so forth.

A distinctive feature of this model is that each division has the necessary support services to undertake its tasks and is responsible for managing those functions. The divisional people in charge of finance, planning, human resources, and so on, report directly to the chiefs of each clinical division. In a matrix design, lateral reporting relationships would also be established with the hospital's vice presidents for finance, planning, human resources, and so on. Divisional designs are currently found in some large teaching hospitals, such as Johns Hopkins Medical Center in Baltimore[7] and Rush-Presbyterian St. Luke's in Chicago.[8]

In a divisional design there is no need for the traditional voluntary medical staff organization because its functions are performed by the clinical divisions themselves and incorporated directly into the line reporting relationships of the hospital. There may be cross-divisional task forces or coordinating committees to handle some organization-wide quality functions or meet accreditation requirements, but the basic organization unit is the division.

A major advantage to the hospital is the ability to better integrate clinical and support services. This may be particularly true under diagnosis related group (DRG)-based prospective payment; divisions could be organized around product/service lines or clusters of given DRGs. By grouping resources within specialized divisions, each group can react more quickly to change its service line as needed. Each group is also directly accountable for managing its resources and for bottom-line financial performance. The Hopkins experience suggests the divisional model can better control resources, improve efficiency, and more flexibly adapt to new payment systems. It may also facilitate the integration and utilization of clinical and administrative data required by new payment systems.

Potential disadvantages to the hospital include the loss of control by administration and, in particular, by the nursing staff. The divisional design decentralizes power, authority, and information to the operating clinical divisions and, in the process, transfers more influence to physicians and support staffs operating those divisions. Such decentralization may be a problem when the hospital faces a number of issues requiring coordination and cooperation across divisions; the more divisions, the greater the problem.

Nursing may oppose divisional designs because of having to report through a physician clinical chief. This was an issue in the Hopkins case, but experience suggests nurses are satisfied with the new design. In particular, they believe they have increased influence and responsibility in patient care and other areas of concern. Further, the quality of communication appears to have improved. Central to this issue is the degree to which the physician clinical/administrative chiefs involve nurses in important patient care and managerial decisions and the relationship between the nursing director and the clinical chief in each division.

The major advantage of the divisional model for physicians is increased authority and control. The physician chief controls all resources needed to provide cost-effective care in the division. Each functional area is contained within the division. In many cases the physician chief reports directly to the president of the hospital, who is often (but need not be) a physician. There is strong physician influence and direction throughout the organization.

A major disadvantage is that not all physicians have the managerial skills, attitudes, or time to make a divisional organization effective. Further, some physicians' work requires close coordination and cooperation across divisions. Strong divisional identity may hinder cross-divisional task performance.

Through the concentration of resources relevant to each division's task, the divisional design can greatly facilitate problem-solving and professional and organizational learning, and promote appropriate risk taking. But the design requires strong physician managers and strong top management to see the larger picture and appropriately coordinate and integrate divisional plans and objectives.

Parallel Model

The third model creates a separate organization to conduct activities not handled well by the formal organization (figure 1.3, next page).[9] Individuals with appropriate skills, experience, and interests are selected to participate. The parallel organization differs from an ad hoc task force or committee because it is intended to be relatively permanent. It differs from a formal matrix design (in which a single person reports to two superiors) because it has no formal dual reporting channels.

The individuals in the parallel organization maintain their operating responsibilities in the formal organization, but some of their time (for example, 25 to 50 percent) is freed up to work in the parallel organization. Often, a steering committee is formed to integrate the ideas of the parallel organization into the formal organization.[10]

The parallel organization deals with major strategic issues facing both the hospital and its medical staff. Examples include hospital-physician joint ventures, new product/service lines, a hospital's teaching responsibilities, and organization-wide productivity and quality. The parallel organization typically involves representatives not only from the medical staff, but also from the nursing staff, other health professions, and administration; expertise, interest, credibility with peers, and interpersonal skills are among the primary criteria for selection. Members are given time off from their daily operating responsibilities and provided with additional compensation to serve in the parallel organization.

A major advantage of the parallel model is its ability to deal with

Figure 1.3. The Parallel Model*

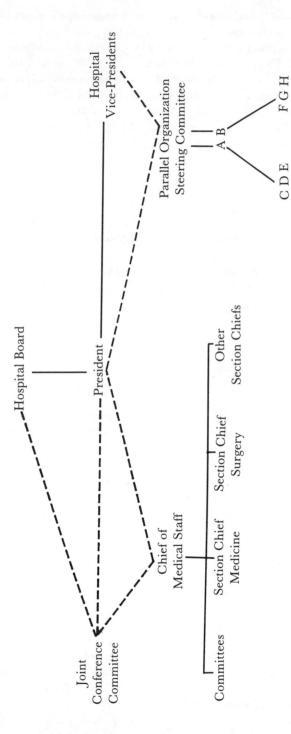

*Individuals in the parallel organization, on the right, are selected from the formal medical staff organization, on the left, and from nursing, other health professions, and administration. In the example shown, individuals A and B serve as coordinators for two subgroups made up of individuals C, D, and E and F, G, and H.

complex, ambiguous, and ill-structured problems not handled well by the current medical staff structure, with its numerous committees and turnover in leadership. It offers a more effective way of involving physicians in managing the organization.

An advantage of the parallel model over the divisional model is that the hospital and its medical staff can deal with organization-wide issues that cut across divisions, thus avoiding potential "balkanization." It also involves a less pervasive change than totally reorganizing along divisional lines. The model permits the traditional medical staff organization to do what it does best: overseeing daily clinical activities. The parallel model's advantage over the independent-corporate model is that it avoids the split of the medical staff from the hospital.

Disadvantages include the start-up time involved, the amount of training and support required, and the danger that the parallel organization might be perceived as a threat by other organization members. These issues must be addressed by committed hospital and medical staff leadership.

For physicians, a major advantage of the parallel model is the opportunity for significant input into issues that affect their long-term interests. The traditional medical staff organization is structured to deal with short-run operational issues. The parallel structure addresses issues relevant to the hospital's long-range plans, involving environmental assessment, competitive analysis, assessment of organizational strengths and weaknesses, and the development of new service lines.

There is an increasing need to involve physicians with appropriate skills, interests, and expertise in all these activities. These physicians may or may not be the formally elected leaders, although communication between the parallel organization and the traditional medical staff is essential. The parallel organization also offers a major advantage in potentially involving younger members of the staff, years before they would usually have the opportunity to play such leadership roles in the traditional medical staff. Thus, the parallel organization can be a vehicle for developing future medical staff leadership.

From the physician's perspective, there are three potential disadvantages: the amount of time involved, the danger that physicians serving in the parallel organization might lose credibility with their peers and become ineffective, and the danger that the parallel organization might usurp some daily operating responsibilities of the medical staff. Time can be addressed by compensation and meaningful involvement. The credibility and usurpation issues can be addressed by appropriate leadership from the steering committee and from the hospital and medical staff.

Hospital/physician PPOs and HMOs are activities that can be undertaken under the parallel model. Ellwood's MeSH plans, separate associations with 50/50 participation of hospitals and physicians, also are an example.[11] St. John's Hospital in Santa Monica has established a separate *associated physicians* organization to deal with alternative delivery systems and related issues.[12] Other hospitals have followed suit. The model developed here goes beyond these examples to incorporate physician input into overall strategic planning and management of the hospital. MeSH plans and physician associations are stepping-stones to a more fully developed parallel model.

The parallel model has major advantages in identifying problems, dealing with ambiguity and change, problem-solving, and developing trust. It is also an excellent forum for "staging" issues, including: (1) anticipating issues for discussion before there is an urgency to resolve them; (2) facing controversial issues far enough in advance so they will seem remote and less threatening; and (3)providing a structure for making decisions.[13] However, the parallel model critically depends on the ability of individual members of the parallel organization to maintain close communication with both the hospital and the formal medical staff.

Criteria for Model Selection

None of the models will fit neatly each hospital's situation. The independent-corporate model may have possibilities where there is a long history of hospital-medical staff conflict, where the hospital is located in a multihospital community, where there is a group of entrepreneurially oriented physicians, and where a number of large multispecialty groups might readily initiate independent medical corporations.

The divisional model may be most appropriate for large, teaching-oriented hospitals with strong clinical divisions, physician managers with experience and expertise, nonphysician executives and managers with the ability to work with professionals, and strong integrating mechanisms across divisions.

The parallel model appears best suited for 200- to 500-bed hospitals with low to moderate teaching activity, operating in a competitive environment, and having a high emphasis on increasing market share for both hospitals and physicians, a strong need for a long-range strategic planning process, credible physician leaders with the necessary time to spend on the issues, and excellent communication links to the traditional medical staff and hospital organization.

The models are not likely to exist in pure form, and mixed models may serve many hospitals' needs. For example, the medical staff may be organized largely along divisional lines, with a parallel organization composed of representatives from each division to work with hospital administration on organization-wide issues.

Another variation would combine the independent-corporate model and the parallel model. In this case, the independent physician corporation and the hospital would name representatives to form a "bipartisan" parallel model for managing ongoing relationships and addressing strategic issues involving the contract between the hospital and the physician corporation. This hybrid might be termed an *integrated-corporate model*.

Although payment mechanisms seem to be moving increasingly toward capitation, hospitals and physicians have considerable freedom to *organize* in ways that promote organizational and professional viability while providing more cost-effective patient care.

These models represent only some of the available choices. Regardless of the choice, a premium will be placed on the ability of hospitals and physicians to communicate, to develop mutual respect and trust, and to actively deal with change and ambiguity. The winners will be those that develop strong hospital-physician partnerships. They will recognize that health care is *both* an economic good and a social good; that physicians will be *both* hospital employees and private practitioners; and that hospitals and physicians will *both* need to compete as well as collaborate.

References

1. Kornhauser, W. *Scientists in Industry.* Berkeley, CA: University of California Press, 1982.
2. Glaser, B. *Organizational Scientists.* Indianapolis: Bobbs-Merrill, 1964.
3. Smith, H. L. Two lines of authority are one too many. *Modern Hospital.* 1955 March. 84:59-64.
4. Shortell, S. M. Patterns of referral among internists and private practice: A social exchange model. *Journal of Health and Social Behavior.* 1973 Dec. 335-348.
5. Shortell, S. M. *A Model of Physician Referral Behavior: A Test of Exchange Theory in Medical Practice,* Research Series, No. 31. Chicago: Center for Health Administration Studies, University of Chicago. December, 1972.
6. Norton D. *Personal Destiny: A Philosophy of Ethical Individualism.* NJ: Princeton University Press, 1976.
7. Heyssel, R. M. The Faculty Role in the Competitive Academic Health Center. Paper delivered at the annual meeting of the Association of Academic Health Centers, Palm Springs, CA, 1981.
8. Sinoris, M. E., Esmond, T. H., and others. The Program Matrix: New Approach to Hospital Planning and Decision-making. Unpublished monograph, Rush-Presbyterian St. Luke's Medical Center, Chicago, IL 1980.
9. Stein, B. A., and Kanter, R. M. Building a parallel organization: Creating mechanisms for permanent quality of work life. *Journal of Applied Behavioral Science.* 1980. 16:371-386.
10. Kanter, R. M. Managing transitions in organizational culture: The case of participative management at Honeywell. In: Kimberly, J., and Quinn, R. (Eds.), *Managing Organizational Transitions.* Homewood, IL: Dow-Jones Irwin, 1984, pp. 195—217.
11. Yanish, D. Hospital work with M.D.'s to smooth MeSH partnerships' rough edges. *Modern Healthcare,* 1984 Feb. 15. 14:58-62.
12. Corlin, R. F. "Healthcare in a Brave New World," Executive Briefing for Hospital Medical Staff Leadership. Creating New Incentives for Physician-Hospital Cooperation, Division of Medical Staff Affairs, American Hospital Association, San Diego, CA, February 23, 1984.
13. Hitt, D. H. Grounding the high intensity in physician-hospital relationships. *Hospitals,* 1984 Apr. 16, 91-95.

Chapter 2
Physicians and Hospitals: Competitors or Partners?

Richard H. Egdahl, M.D., and Cynthia H. Taft, M.A.

Hospital-medical staff relationships are receiving much attention lately because both physicians and the hospitals they admit patients to are facing new constraints and challenges. In order to understand how both parties will respond, it is important to consider several fundamental questions first.

- What will be the basic role of the hospital in the future?
- What are the areas of cooperation between the hospital and its medical staff?
- What are areas of potential competition between the two?
- What is the appropriate corporate relationship between hospital and medical staff?
- What will be the impact of competitive health plans on both the hospital and its medical staff?

The answers to these questions depend upon the kind of health care delivery system that emerges from the current economic, political, and social climate. One scenario will unfold if most physicians in the future are salaried and if health maintenance organizations (HMOs) become the dominant mode of medical practice. A different set of relationships will develop if fee-for-service with rigorous utilization review continues to be the principal mode of practice and if preferred provider arrangements (PPAs) involving mostly fee-for-service practice grow more rapidly than HMOs.

The Hospital of the Future

Will the hospital assume a larger role in coming years by managing the majority of the health care delivery system. Or will it continue to be the focus of care for patients needing special resources and treatment?

The answer depends on whether individual hospitals become complete

Dr. Egdahl is Director, Boston University Medical Center, Boston, MA.

Ms. Taft is Vice-President for Clinical Operations, New England Medical Center, Boston, MA.

health care delivery systems or continue to function primarily as enterprises providing a principal product: inpatient care. Many hospitals have embarked on new business activities by establishing holding companies that can develop for-profit ventures and by joining multi-institutional systems that are launching ventures. These activities include a wide range of health care delivery services, including ambulatory and surgical centers, nursing homes, and home health care services.

Despite diversification efforts, however, the major goal of hospitals remains the same: the economic and professional survival and growth of the hospital. CEOs hope that surpluses from profitable new ventures (such as home health care, pharmacies, and real estate transactions) will subsidize intrinsically nonprofitable ones (such as education and care of the poor). Thus, it seems unlikely that their new ventures will become the prime focus of most community or teaching hospitals, as we know them today. Their central mission will continue to be to care for patients who cannot be treated on an ambulatory basis or at home. However, hospitals will participate increasingly in joint marketing ventures to expand their market share, fill beds, and increase revenues.

Areas of Hospital-Medical Staff Cooperation

There are several areas where hospital-medical staff cooperation is necessary, desirable, and relatively easy to achieve.

Credentialing and Privileges

Although it is the ultimate responsibility of hospital trustees to approve appointments to the medical staff, the review of credentials and definition of specific privileges must be carried out by clinicians able to assess the training and clinical experience of medical staff applicants. But hospital management and trustees may want to set targets for the number of practicing specialists. They may choose to do this for several reasons, including the need for surgeons to perform a critical mass of certain surgical procedures in order to retain their competence. Determining the appropriate number and mix of hospital staff physicians is a function that only trustees—with outside advice—can perform. Otherwise, the medical staff faces potential antitrust violations if it makes decisions that could limit competition.

Quality of Care

Another area of cooperation centers around quality care issues. This cooperation is important to prevent not only overutilization but the possibility of underutilization, as a result of the strong financial incentives in primary care gatekeeper systems and managed care health plans. It is in the best interests of both hospitals and physicians that quality of care be rigorously monitored. And both hospital managers and physicians should be included in the development of these programs.

Capital Expenditures

With respect to capital budgets, management will continue to retain ulti-mate decision-making authority. But active professional input is necessary if capital expenditures are to match clinical priorities. Key clinicians must be deeply involved in the ongoing strategic planning process that matches financial resources with expected patient activity.

Marketing

A major thrust for all hospitals in the future will be marketing their products, in the broadest sense. Strong collaboration between hospital management and clinicians is necessary in order to define the primary products, to develop a strategy for marketing these products effectively to physician users and consumers, and, thus, to expand the hospital's market share. In this latter goal, the interests of physicians and hospital management should most completely coincide.

Areas of Potential Competition

There are also several areas of potential hospital-medical staff competition. Payments to hospitals based on diagnosis-related groups (DRGs) or other global norms may lead to potential conflicts. Hospitals have incentives to shorten lengths of stay in a given DRG, whereas physicians are usually paid by patient days spent in the hospital. Thus, an internist taking care of a patient with a complicated medical disorder currently has every incentive to hospitalize that patient as long as he or she believes it to be medically advisable. The physician's personal financial incentive is also for continued hospitalization, as he or she is paid a fee for each day the patient spends in the hospital. On the other hand, the hospital would fare better financially if the patient were discharged earlier, provided it is medically feasible.

There are also potential conflicts when the hospital is paid a flat rate for the treatment of patients with specific diseases. This can occur either with capitation, DRGs, or HMO contracts. For example, a patient may need to have cardiac catheterization and open-heart surgery. The capitating vehicle, HMO, or DRG payer wants to pay some entity a single lump sum, combin-ing all private professional fees and hospital charges. Hospitals and practic-ing physicians must then agree on how to share this global payment.

Another area of potential competition exists when hospitals decide to build and manage centers that offer ambulatory surgery, emergency, or primary care services. Hospitals and their medical staffs occasionally develop joint ventures to carry out these activities. But such ventures may still compete with the practices of nonparticipating physician members of the medical staff.

Underlying this potential area of competition are basic questions relating to the hospital's role. According to Paul Ellwood, Jr., M.D., "Hospitals are in a new business. . .the business of practicing medicine."[1] And John Witt, president of Witt and Associates, Oak Brook, IL, claims that "hospitals are losing the advantage which the physician surplus has created for them, and should be hiring physicians as employees, not playing into physicians' hands by preserving the private practice system."[2] If so, will physician medical staffs in the future be hospital employees or private practitioners of medicine?

The best evidence suggests that physicians will continue to practice as independent professionals, and hospitals will continue to compete for the best and most efficient physicians to staff their facilities. For example, in the case of national networks being developed to deliver care to large employer organizations, such as the Voluntary Hospitals of America/Aetna plans and Humana's Care Plus, physicians are not regarded as employees of the hospitals of management corporations. They are looked upon as private practitioners, even though there are strong financial incentives to hospitalize patients in plan hospitals. There currently is no trend towards "hiring" doctors as employees of these hospital systems (or of most other hospitals, with a few exceptions).

Corporate Structures for Joint Ventures

Hospital-medical staff relationships are complex because physicians function both as medical staff members and as private practitioners. However, the medical staff needs a corporate vehicle for its independent physicians to engage in joint ventures with its hospital. These can take one of three forms. First, the hospital may be an employer. This form appears unlikely to gain strength in the future, although some experts have suggested that it may become a trend. Another way is for the hospital to be the dominant partner in a joint venture with physicians. This corporate vehicle will probably turn out to be divisive in most instances, as there will be a jockeying for power and some physicians will be left out.

The model with the best chance of working, in the authors' view, is separate hospital and medical staff corporations. Under this model, the medical staff corporation takes private practice revenues and redistributes them according to formulas worked out among the various groups and individual practitioners on the medical staff. Figure 2.1, next page, illustrates a way in which global payments could be received by a joint committee of the hospital and medical staff corporations. The joint committee

Figure 2.1. Process for Distributing Global Payments under a Hospital-Medical Staff Joint Venture

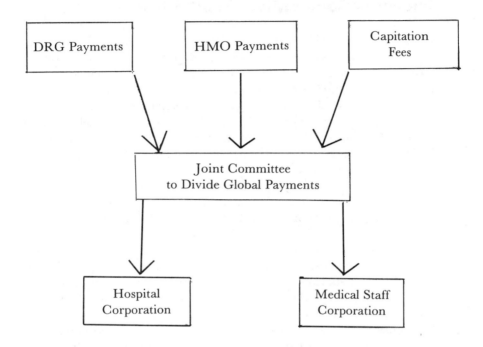

would divide the payments into two components, then the medical staff and hospital corporations would decide how to use those funds to fulfill their contract for services.

Impact of Competitive Health Plans

A radical change is under way in terms of how hospitals are paid. Payment is now based on illness or some other category rather than on costs, as in the past. What is not as generally understood, however, is that an equally radical change is under way in terms of how efficiently physicians practice medicine. This development is prompting dialogues between the hospital management and the medical staff on how they can work together to shorten lengths of stay or order fewer laboratory tests without compromising the health of patients, thereby saving the hospital money and freeing up resources for other critical needs.

Managed care health plans, sponsored by a wide variety of competing insurers, are leading directly to major changes in practice routines. They are providing the necessary stimulus for the survival of personalized fee-for-service practice, albeit in a considerably more efficient form. Physicians are changing their practice routines because (1) rigorous utilization control conditions are built into managed health benefit plans, and (2) they need patients and are in danger of losing their share in an increasingly competitive practice world. Managed health care plans benefit financially from greater practice efficiency, because they pay only for the hospital days, laboratory tests, and admissions utilized by their covered population. Hospitals, on the other hand, are put under financial pressure from these plans because greatly shortened lengths of stay have an impact on occupancy, and hospitals are left with the more intense and expensive days of care.

Examples of the pressures managed care health plans and successful individual practice associations (IPAs) are exerting on physicians are numerous. The Pilgrim Health Care plan, an IPA in southeastern Massachusetts, recently sent out a new instruction to physician members, which read: "We must insist that all patients be admitted for elective surgery on the same day the surgery is performed."[3] Bay State Health Care, an IPA in the Boston area, has stipulated, "All elective inpatient surgical admissions are to be scheduled for surgery on the day of admission unless specifically exempted." The Bay State Health Care plan also states, "Beginning with referred services provided on June 1, 1985, referral providers must have a written referral from the patient's designated primary care physician." Bay State has also ruled, "All claims should be submitted within 30 days following the date of service,"[4] and the IPA can suspend payment if claims are submitted after more than 90 days. It is quite clear that adherence to these principles will result in greatly decreased lengths of stay, rapid submission of claims, and fewer casual referrals to consultant specialists.

Health plans are also using strong financial incentives to reduce utilization of hospital days and medical treatments. For example, United States Health Care System, Inc., a rapidly growing profit-making HMO, based in Pennsylvania, is structured so that primary care gatekeepers benefit financially from less-than-customary hospitalizations and less use of specialists. In the Met-Elect program, a preferred provider plan of the Dade County (FL) School System, physicians are picked for their efficiency, based on claims data. Patients pay a 20 percent copayment if they do not use the plan and need approval of a Met-Elect staff nurse before hospitalization.

Mounting pressures to improve practice efficiency are increasingly reflected in the medical literature. For example, R. C. Hall, M.D., Metro-Health Plan, Indianapolis, has published his results with cholecystectomy patients. Dr. Hall admits most patients two hours before surgery and discharges them about two days later.[5] The most efficient routine cholecystectomy is performed by Gerald Moss, M.D., of Rensselaer Polytecnic Institute, Troy, NY. Dr. Moss hospitalizes his patients for an average of 1.0 + 1 day. He achieves this result by administering a full-strength elemental diet by a small tube in the recovery room and using local anesthetics in the wound before closure. His patients are informed preoperatively that they will be leaving the hospital on the first postoperative day unless complications occur.[6]

Irving Lichtenstein, M.D., Los Angeles, has published his experiences with hernia patients over many years. Most of his patients leave the hospital within one day of surgery. Ninety percent receive no injections for pain, and skin clips are out within 24 hours of surgery. Currently, most of his patients are operated on as outpatients.[7]

The Duke University Hospital cardiology group has also shown that approximately half of patients with myocardial infarction do not have complications by the seventh hospital day and can be safely discharged.[8] More recently, a report from Jackson Memorial Hospital, Miami, describes how 10 changes in routines in the surgical intensive care unit (ICU) resulted in 42 percent fewer laboratory tests and 53 percent fewer ICU laboratory charges. Extrapolating these results to one year's population in the 12-bed surgical ICU brought about a $2 million reduction in charges.[9]

A growing body of literature thus indicates that efficient practice routines can be obtained under special circumstances, without apparent loss in quality of care. These experiences, combined with the pressures of managed care and prepaid health care plans, make it clear that practice patterns will be pushed hard in the future toward the margin of what could be called "undercare." The PSRO program was largely set up to decrease overcare and bring practice patterns into the "acceptable" area. We are now rapidly moving through the acceptable range of care toward undercare, which will require more subtle forms of review than mortality and morbidity indexes.

Overcare, experts agree, exists when normal gallbladders are removed, when herniorrhaphy is carried out for an impulse (but not a hernia) in the inguinal ring, and when patients are hospitalized for a low-grade fever and diarrhea, without an ambulatory workup. Falling within the acceptable range of care today are removal of a solid thyroid nodule, hysterectomy for fibroids with repeated bleeding, hospitalization of patients with mild diabetic acidosis, and a preoperative hospital day for major elective surgery. But these currently acceptable standards will undergo pressures from the financial incentives built into health care plans.

Underutilization of health services will soon be a key concern, and procedures must evolve to identify it. For example, a premature discharge evaluation protocol might specify indicators of premature discharge or inadequate discharge planning and be predictive of adverse postdischarge patient outcomes. Indicators for adverse postdischarge patient outcomes might be readmission to the hospital, a new admission to a nursing home, lowered functional status, or death.

Summary

In the future of hospital-medical staff relationships, hospitals will be used only when absolutely necessary, because of their high cost compared to the ambulatory setting. This will lead to the need to focus on undercare as a potential major problem.

Hospitals and their medical staffs will cooperate in marketing to get patients, in decisions on capital budgets, in credentialing of physicians for hospital privileges, and in quality of care area issues, especially undercare. Hospitals and their medical staffs will also compete in some cases. Physicians will not become employees of most hospitals, but fee-for-service practices and salaried group practices will compete, with the survivors being those who practice most efficiently. Hospitals and their medical staffs will need separate corporations to work together and divide and allocate capitation, HMO, or DRG payments.

References

1. Doctor cooperation needed under PPS. *Hospitals.* 1984 Mar.1. 58(5):26.
2. Richman, D. Hospital-staff ventures popular, but critics question their worth. *Modern Healthcare.* 1985 May 24. 15(11):80-81.
3. *Pilgrim Health Care IPA News Brief.* Office of the Medical Director. June 1, 1985, p. 1.
4. *Bay State Health Care Prospects.* 1985 June. 2(4):2.
5. Hall, R. Patient acceptance of admission two hours before and discharge two days after cholecystectomy. In: *HMOs in the Mainstream: Sustaining Growth and Equality.* 1983 Group Health Institute Proceedings, June 12, 1983, pp. 103-15.
6. Moss, G., Regal, M., and Lichtig, L. Reducing postoperative pain, narcotics, and length of hospitalization. *Surgery.* 1986 Feb. 99(2):206-10.
7. Lichtenstein, I. L. Modern advances in hernia surgery. Part 1: The 'one day' inguinal herniorrhaphy. *Contemporary Surgery.* 1982 Apr. 20:17-36.

8. McNeer, J. F., Wagner, G. S., and others. Hospital discharge one week after acute myocardial infarction. *New England Journal of Medicine* 1978 Feb. 2. 298(5):229-32.
9. Civetta, J. M., and Hudson-Civetta, J. A. Maintaining quality of care while reducing charges in the ICU. *Annals of Surgery.* 1985 Oct. 202(4):524-30.

Chapter 3

The Joint Venture Phenomenon: A Response to Sweeping Change

Steven Landgarten, M.D.

Heightened joint venture activity between hospitals and their medical staffs is a product of changing times. Both hospitals and physicians are facing excess capacity and numbers, new reimbursement schemes, and the need to better control patient flow.

To be sure, joint economic activity raises new liability concerns, potential conflicts with corporate practices of medicine acts, and competitive fears among some medical staff members. But the benefits of hospitals and their medical staffs banding together in new partnerships continue to fuel the joint venture trend. Among those benefits are immediate tax advantages for physicians, reduced capital requirements for hospitals, better long-term control over patient flow, and relief of some long-standing stresses and strains in the traditional hospital-medical staff relationship.

The Changing Nature of Hospitals

Recent changes in hospital operations and the physician environment have largely prompted the flurry of joint ventures. In the hospital sector, for example, prospective pricing has drastically altered how hospitals generate more revenue. Traditionally, most hospitals expanded revenue by increasing the volume and sophistication of services provided to their existing patient base. Market share was less important than patient mix and the volume of ancillary services. Indeed, hospitals enhanced revenue in much the same way automobile dealers improve profits by adding ''mandatory options,'' rather than increasing the number of cars sold. However, this technique no longer applies to the growing cohort of patients covered by various prospective payment systems.

Prospective pricing, and the economic forces that originally led to prospective systems, are also causing a shift from inpatient to outpatient care. The volume of inpatient services provided by hospitals is therefore declining, and inpatient dollars are becoming a shrinking proportion of gross institutional revenue.

Dr. Landgarten is Vice-President for Medical Affairs, Hillcrest Medical Center, Tulsa, OK.

With fewer inpatients and inpatient dollars, hospitals are being forced to compete for shares of an ever-shrinking market. Not only are hospitals competing with each other at the local level, but with regional referral centers as well. To survive, many are joining noncompetitors in systems and alliances, several of which are launching insurance products to attract new business. A number of hospitals that have chosen to remain independent are finding it difficult to compete with such integrated systems.

The advent of diagnosis-related groups (DRGs) has given hospitals on the system the opportunity to engage in nonoperating revenue activity. Previously, any source of revenue that was not sheltered by restrictions and board-designated limitations, either philanthropic or through health-related business ventures, was calculated in cost-based reimbursement and, in essence, functioned as a subsidy to the Medicare program rather than as a bottom-line benefit to the institution. Under systems of prospective payment, additional revenues gained though various business ventures produce a more favorable financial impact on the institution.

The Changing Physician Environment

Many of the same forces that have changed hospitals have had an impact on physicians. Just as hospitals must cope with overcapacity, so physicians are experiencing a surplus in their numbers. In most large and medium-sized communities, the physician population has risen faster than the general population, effectively reducing market share. Indeed, most national surveys have documented a reduction in annual patient visits per physician as well as revenue per physician. In addition to market share reduction, physicians are being subjected to new payment constraints that have an impact on their revenue stream. Constraints in the public sector include a freeze on Medicare reimbursement, a freeze on Medicaid reimbursement in many states, and the threat of a federal prospective or mandatory assignment system of physician reimbursement. Additionally, in the private sector growing numbers of patients are enrolling in preferred provider arrangements (PPAs), which may reduce fees directly as well as require stringent utilization review.

Just as hospitals that function independently and not as part of a network are at a marketing disadvantage today, so solo practitioners lack the marketing clout and control over patient flow that their colleagues participating in PPAs enjoy. As a result, independent physicians are allying themselves more closely with hospitals, health maintenance organizations (HMOs), and other entities. The number of physicians who have established employment or contractual relationships with health care institutions has risen to 25 percent, by some estimates.[1] More physicians are also opting for the security of a salaried position with an HMO rather than the independence and risk of a solo practice.

The Traditional Hospital-Medical Staff Relationship

The move toward a more competitive environment and, with it, an increase in joint venture activity are being superimposed on a hospital-medical staff relationship that has evolved over the course of 40 years. In the process, constraints imposed by the present structure are becoming evident, as well as the need for change if both hospitals and their medical staffs are to evolve toward a new system of partnerships.

Traditionally, the organized medical staff has represented individual entrepreneurship. Responsibilities that hospitals delegated to the medical staff, which it provided as a service, were honored only as long as they did not limit that entrepreneurship. Indeed, in many situations, physician ego and economics have been protected at the expense of institutional interests. In extreme circumstances, these interests have been protected even at the expense of the community.

Besides delegated responsibilities, hospitals themselves have been viewed ambivalently by physicians. Although hospitals have provided physicians with the tools of production, they have also regulated physician activity and, increasingly, become potential competitors for the provision of services. For these reasons, as well as the impact hospital policy has on the provision of health care in a community, many physicians would now like a strong role in institutional policy. Up to this time, physicians have felt that their input into institutional policy has been inadequate in many situations.

Hospitals, in turn, have generally viewed the medical staff as an asset to be managed. But managing this asset is difficult and entails the close cooperation of the medical staff itself. For example, hospitals have accepted accountability for the quality of medical services and of the medical staff, but they can carry it out only through delegation to the medical staff members. Moreover, while medical staff mix is critical to the hospital in terms of providing an adequate spectrum of services, that mix is extremely difficult to control. In most situations, physicians are far more easily recruited by other physicians than by the institution itself.

A new area of potential conflict in perspective between hospitals and their medical staffs is prospective pricing systems. Under these systems, hospitals have important financial incentives to curb the number of services per patient stay. Physicians are concerned lest some institutions do so at the expense of quality of medical care.

The Value of Joint Ventures

Joint ventures provide a number of solutions to the real and potential conflicts and concerns outlined earlier. Hospitals stand to gain in major ways. Most health care "futurists" maintain that controlling patient flow is the key to future survival for health care organizations. The hospitals that will survive, then, will be integrated systems that include both inpatient and outpatient providers, primary and specialized care, elements of geographic dispersion, and, possibly, an insurance product linking the individual elements. Such integrated organizations have already emerged in both the not-for-profit and investor-owned sectors.

In addition to clear institutional benefits, joint ventures offer distinct advantages to hospitals in their relationship with the medical staff. Most obvious of course, is mutual financial benefit. The benefit may be as simple as physicians gaining tax advantages and the hospital reducing its need for capital.

But other, more subtle, benefits may also emerge. Within the legal structure of partnerships formed for such activities as surgicenters, diagnostic centers, convenient care practices, and other physician-based activities, the partners, including physicians, may well assume a corporate obligation to provide quality assurance and other services heretofore supplied on a strictly "voluntary" basis by the organized medical staff. Under this framework, physician egos will be protected only at the expense of *physician* economics. This is in stark contrast to the all too frequent circumstance within organized medical staffs in which physician egos are protected at the expense of hospital economics. As one hospital administrator put it at a joint venture board meeting, "Doctor, welcome to the real world."

Under a joint venture structure, many of the participating physicians may come to view the hospital as a true partner, rather than a regulator or even adversary. Joint ventures also superimpose an enforced joint responsibility for quality and policy development. Thus, a hospital and medical staff with multiple joint ventures between them will probably evolve into a better health care organization than those that preserve the traditional separation of hospital and medical staff affairs.

Models of Joint Ventures

Although joint ventures have become quite popular in the last several years and have received considerable publicity, in reality they are not new. For at least the past 15 years, many community hospitals have sponsored physician office buildings. That sponsorship has been direct, through a shared investment with physicians, or indirect, through hospital capitalization of the project as a form of subsidy to encourage physicians to practice nearby. This is the "traditional" form of joint venture.

Newer forms have emerged over the past five to seven years. Those that appear to be growing most rapidly are freestanding surgicenters, general diagnostic imaging centers, and selective diagnostic centers, including magnetic resonance imaging, mammography, sports medicine, and similar "storefront" activities. There has also been a proliferation of urgent or convenience care centers. These centers are established either singly, as a venture between an individual physician or physician group and the hospital, or as part of a geographically dispersed network, with other institutions. One voluntary hospital in the Midwest has established a series of six centers and strategically located them so as to enhance its attractiveness to HMOs and other alternate care providers, as well as to provide well-defined market salients in traditional referral areas of competing hospitals.

Joint ventures involving convenient care centers must be handled with caution, however. In launching such centers, the hospital may be assuming, for the first time, corporate responsibility for the quality of care rendered in essentially a private practice clinical site. Previously, the hospital's liability was limited to the care rendered within its own walls. The hospital's medical staff must therefore closely supervise care in the centers by establishing medical care standards, as well as an organized review of the quality of care rendered there. Both the hospital and medical staff must ensure that the quality of care delivered in the centers does not vary from that expected within the hospital itself.

Liability for the quality of medical care is not the only risk in this type of venture. In many communities, hospital involvement in convenient care centers has been viewed as unfair competition by some members of the medical staff. The choice of sites for these centers is therefore critical. The establishment of a center that competes directly with a primary care practice that has always been supportive of the hospital is not in anyone's best interest.

Sensitive policy decisions that distinguish between episodic and ongoing care, and define the convenient care center's purview, must also be made. A center that sees patients only on an episodic basis and refers those in need of follow-up to primary care physicians is supportive of the traditional medical staff structure. Centers that invite patients to return for follow-up, and even continuing care, may be more economically successful as a joint venture, but more disruptive of traditional medical staff relationships.

Many other clinical services are also being offered on a joint venture basis. These include cancer treatment centers, dialysis centers, and joint home health care programs. In some of the latter, the organized medical staff or a multispecialty clinic, or both, form a joint venture with a partner experienced in the provision of home health care, durable medical equipment, or home oxygen. Several prototypes of this kind of joint venture exist on the West Coast and are emerging as economically successful.

A more intimate relationship develops between a hospital and its medical staff when they engage in joint practice activities. These joint ventures include private practice development or purchase, or group practice management and development for the provision of direct management services, including practice marketing to individual and group members of the medical staff through a jointly owned and operated medical practice subsidiary. Before embarking on such ventures, hospitals and physicians should evaluate corporate practice of medicine acts in their state.

On a larger scale, many hospitals are joint venturing with their medical staffs or large multispecialty groups within their staffs to establish alternate provider systems and networks. The models include medical staff PPAs, medical staff-based independent practice associations, group model HMOs, and regional provider networks of both the PPA and HMO type.

Building Consensus and Support

Hospitals often set about the joint venture process by trying to decide, "What joint venture should we tackle first?" But some important groundwork needs to precede that decision. Hospitals should concentrate initially on fostering an environment supportive of innovation and change, starting with the medical staff.

Assessing the nature and needs of the medical staff involved is critical. Every staff has within it competitors and noncompetitors, risk-takers and traditionalists, old and young. Each of these groups has its own perspective on specific ventures, as well as on the concept of hospitals entering into joint economic relationships with physicians to deliver medical care.

To create an environment receptive to change, the hospital must bring these diverse groups to a common understanding of joint ventures, how they fit into its mission, and how they will contribute to its financial viability. This requires a process of "desensitization," during which concerns and fears are diffused, questions are answered, and substantial information and education are provided.

The educational process should build consensus among the medical staff for the idea of joint ventures in general. But physicians must also understand that not every venture proposed will be attractive to all, or even a majority, of them. As hospital managers suggest ideas for ventures, small groups of interested physicians will identify themselves. Then, it is up to the hospital to actively support and encourage their entrepreneurial involvement.

When the joint venture parties sit down to structure their new business, hospital managers should realize that physicians' motivations often differ substantially from their own. Most physicians are strongly motivated by independence and, through their training, have developed a primary commitment to their patients, rather than aggregate institutional or social goals. The motivating force of ego and economics should also be considered in structuring a venture.

Reference

1. Reynolds, Roger A., and Ohsfeldt, Robert L., eds. *Socioeconomic Characteristics of Medical Practice.* Chicago: American Medical Association, 1984.

Chapter 4

The Medical Staff Role in Health Care Networks

Penelope C. Roeder, M.B.A., and John H. Moxley, III, M.D.

Since the 1983 introduction of the prospective payment system (PPS) for Medicare inpatient hospitalization, the American health care delivery system has been undergoing significant change. That transformation is not yet complete. As the diagnosis-related group (DRG) system is modified and expanded, as capitated systems are developed, and as public-sector models are adapted by the private sector, the restructuring will continue. Throughout this process, the hospital's role in the health care system will also continue to change. With these changes, the needs and demands of medical staffs will shift as well. By understanding some of the forces that are shaping these changes in health care and some of the issues they raise, it may be possible to guide developments toward a more effective health delivery system.

Networking Defined

Current relationships within and among various constituencies of the health care system vary widely. Whether these relationships take the form of preferred provider arrangements (PPAs), health maintenance organizations (HMOs), or freestanding ambulatory centers, they are part of an overall strategy often referred to as *vertical integration*. More accurately, they are examples of *bundling* or *product integration*. It is this ''product integration—the common ownership or control of enterprises that produce distinctly different, but related, products or services''[1]—that is often described as networking.

Networking strategies have been adopted by a wide variety of hospitals— not-for-profit, investor-owned, system-affiliated, and freestanding. There are, to be sure, differences in the legal structures and financing mechanisms available to different organizations, and there has been some variation in the pace at which the strategies have been adopted. However, most product integration efforts have been in response to external factors that affect

Ms. Roeder is Director, Corporate Planning, American Medical International, Inc., Beverly Hills, CA.

Dr. Moxley is Senior Vice-President, American Medical International, Inc., Beverly Hills, CA.

virtually all hospitals, regardless of ownership. Many of these environmental forces are, themselves, the natural by-products of previous changes in the health and hospital system.

Hospitals in Health Care before PPS

The history of general acute care hospitals generally parallels the histories of surgery and medical education. Prior to the development of aseptic surgical techniques at the end of the 19th century, surgery was performed wherever it was most convenient, often at home. Hospitals were, in large measure, places for the sick poor—as much in order to contain disease as for the provision of care.

By the early 20th century, the development of both surgical technique and an organized clinical curriculum for medical students made it more convenient for physicians to deliver increasing amounts of patient care in hospitals. In addition, it was more efficient to administer postoperative care to a number of patients simultaneously. As the use of both diagnostic testing and surgery continued to expand into the midcentury, so did the reliance on institutional care.

A number of economic developments reinforced the growing use of hospitals. First, as physicians began to admit their private patients to hospitals, hospital administrators recognized that private fees represented a potential source of revenues to support the institutions' charitable missions. Then, as hospitals became a more common—as well as a more expensive— place to treat the sick, hospital care came to be viewed as a shared responsibility of the community. Thus, Blue Cross hospital insurance evolved in the early 1930s in order to ensure both the preservation of hospitals and care for the entire community by spreading financial risk. Community rating was introduced as an important insurance principle, which lasted until the late 1970s.

The Growth of Health Insurance

Coverage under these early hospital insurance policies did not include physician services. Physicians had fought hard against insurance for the same basic reason some now fight network arrangements: fear of disruption in the direct physician-patient relationship. Some years later, the physician-controlled Blue Shield Association did introduce insurance to cover physician services. The new policies provided coverage for hospital-related physician services only. In addition, they indemnified patients for physician fees, instead of making direct payment to physicians as Blue Cross did to hospitals. The overall intent was to provide financial insurance for the patient without altering the physician-patient relationship.

After World War II, tax benefits contributed to the spread of health insurance as an employee benefit, and, in 1965, Social Security was expanded to include Medicare, a health insurance plan for the nation's elderly. Most of the insurance plans developed throughout this period of rapid growth were modeled on the first Blue Cross/Blue Shield plan. Although major medical coverage usually included physician and other professional services, most plans focused on hospital care and provided better coverage for inpatient than ambulatory services. In general, that arrangement suited physicians, who increasingly found it more efficient to do hospital rounds than to make house calls.

Throughout the 1950s and 1960s, economics, technology, and physician convenience worked together to make "health care" synonymous with "hospital care" in the public's mind. Yet, there was an irony in that public perception: most health care was, in fact, delivered and controlled by physicians.

Pervasive physician influence has always existed at smaller hospitals. In some cases, small community facilities were started by groups of physicians who pooled their own resources or sought out investors to buy equipment and hire personnel to help care for patients. The Hill-Burton Act (1946) was specifically designed to finance the construction of facilities that would attract physicians to medically underserved communities. These historical antecedents contributed to a view of hospitals as "doctors' workshops." In this context, hospital administrations were often viewed—and viewed themselves—as managing the facility on behalf of the physicians who used it.

This relationship between hospital administration and the medical staff has not been obvious at hospitals with university and medical school affiliations. These institutions have traditionally had a variety of missions. They have, thus, been affected by their particular community's values regarding charity and philanthropy, as well as by the politics and economics of education and research. In addition, medical school hospitals have always had a relatively large number of salaried physicians. However, the dominance of physicians in these hospitals has been manifest in the influence generally exercised by medical school departments on hospital policy and investment decisions.[2]

A More Explicit Relationship

The creation of Medicare, with its cost-based reimbursement policies that resulted in more predictable cash flows, allowed hospitals to enter the public money markets. It thus contributed to making the economic relationship between hospitals and their medical staffs more explicit. Previously, community support and philanthropy had depended, in part, on how physicians viewed the facility and how the public perceived the medical staff. By the mid-1970s, however, hospital survival could, and often did, depend explicitly on physician use. By then, government funds and philanthropy provided only a small and decreasing portion of the total capital needed. The primary sources of funds were patient revenues and debt, and the availability and/or cost of debt often depended heavily on utilization and patient revenues.

At the same time, however, physicians were becoming more independent of hospitals. Much of what had been hospital practice in earlier decades was increasingly becoming office practice. Health planning legislation had begun forcing hospitals and their medical staffs to examine capital expenditures, and certificate-of-need regulations often made it difficult for them to acquire new equipment. As a result, hospitals were occasionally barred from adding new technologies. Many of these new technologies centered on noninvasive diagnostics or other procedures that could be delivered to outpatients, often in a nonhospital setting. Physicians, who were not affected by most planning regulations, therefore began to incorporate the new technologies into their practices by purchasing their own equipment for office use. Thus began the trend away from the practice of treating all patients in the hospital.

Although technological developments in the 1970s encouraged the expansion of both hospital outpatient and freestanding out-of-hospital services, health insurance plans did not generally keep pace with these changes. Medicare and most commercial plans tended to favor inpatient over outpatient treatment, despite the fact that patients increasingly appreciated the convenience of outpatient and out-of-hospital services. Thus, physician facilities were increasingly used for elective procedures such as plastic surgery, which were not well-covered by most insurance, or for contracted procedures such as lab work and X rays.

There was little economic tension between hospitals and their medical staffs during this period. As long as Medicare paid for inpatient care on a cost basis and most commercial insurers paid hospital charges, hospitals could still lose some patients to out-of-hospital services and make up for lost income by raising prices or providing additional services to remaining inpatients. In many instances, both the out-of-hospital services and additional inpatient services generated incremental revenue for physicians who provided the patient care. Thus, the expansion of medical technologies and the growth of out-of-hospital services tended to benefit all constituencies by encouraging the use of additional services for all patients.

The Seeds of Economic Tension

Although major economic conflict between hospitals and physicians did not erupt during the early years of Medicare, its seeds were sown. Hospitals were forced not only to develop some business-like systems and attitudes to adapt to the demands of the public money markets but also to be increasingly responsive to physician demands in order to encourage continued utilization. That responsiveness was heightened, to some extent, by the widespread perception of a physician shortage. At the same time, health planning regulations forced both hospitals and physicians to rethink their capital investment plans. New technologies suitable for outpatient use and increasing physician entrepreneurship encouraged medical staff members to develop alternative sites of care. Only the fact that the medical care system was essentially an open economic system—virtually devoid of risk—permitted the stability between physicians and hospitals that existed between the passage of Medicare and the introduction of DRGs.

By the late 1970s, stability within the health care system extended only as far as relations among providers. The public was becoming increasingly aware of, and discontented with, the nation's growing health care bill. Under Presidents Nixon and Carter, some initiatives to curb those expenditures had been launched. There was, however, no attempt to change the fundamental economics of the reimbursement system until the Reagan Administration demanded that Medicare budget growth be slowed. The private sector, burdened by both continuing recessionary pressures on profits and rapidly increasing health insurance premiums, also sought to end rising health care costs. With such widespread support, Congress was able to introduce the DRG-based prospective payment system in 1983.

Prospective Payment and the Growth of Networks

Along with prospective payment and DRGs came economic risk. DRGs also brought about an abrupt realignment in health insurance priorities: suddenly, limitations were applied to inpatient care and incentives introduced for outpatient care. As private-sector health insurers began to make similar changes, the once open economic system of health care became increasingly closed. Conflict between interdependent physician and hospital competitors began to erupt, often with a force that would radically change the nature of the health care system.

Initially, the introduction of inpatient DRGs forced hospitals to view their traditional inpatient acute care function as part of a much broader health care delivery system. Given the previous decade's development of out-of-hospital services by physicians, this new role threatened to create massive economic problems for hospitals. In order to retain patients who would now receive care in a variety of settings, hospitals had to control those alternative sites. They had two choices: they could expand their own outpatient services, and often directly compete with members of their medical staffs, or they could develop joint ventures with their medical staffs.

Problems in Joint Venture Development

The same cost containment impetus that had led to the introduction of DRGs often made the development of hospital-physician joint ventures difficult. Frequently, during negotiations, the parties became increasingly aware that they were economic competitors vis-a-vis outpatient services.

Even if they could agree upon the financial structure of the venture, deciding where to locate the freestanding facility was complex. If the facility was too close to the hospital, the hospital risked losing income from its own outpatient services. If the facility was built as a satellite to attract new patients from a competitive hospital, the hospital partner might lose inpatient admissions to the competitor based on patient convenience.

During this period, the issue of patient convenience began to assume new and troubling proportions for hospitals, which continued to derive most of their income from inpatient care. Although few physicians had been heedless of patient desires in the past, the limitations on care imposed by both the DRGs and new private health insurance constraints—coupled with the growing number of medical school graduates—encouraged many physicians to become more responsive to their patients' wants. Otherwise, they could lose those patients to physicians who appeared to be more responsive. Thus, an additional limitation of freestanding outpatient joint ventures soon became apparent: since the physicians and the hospital shared economic interests only with regard to the joint venture, the hospital partner could lose potentially profitable inpatient cases if patients demanded, and physicians offered, outpatient treatment.

Facility-Oriented Ventures

In order to counter this tendency for physicians to behave as competitors to the hospital, some institutions—both not-for-profit and investor-owned—have begun to develop joint ventures that focus on the inpatient institution. In some of these ventures, members of the medical staff and the hospital itself become shareholders in a separately incorporated for-profit subsidiary that owns the hospital. As an alternative to these joint ownership arrangements (often referred to as MeSHs), some hospitals have developed arrangements whereby fees are prepaid to physicians who admit a high number of patients.[3]

Although facility-oriented joint ventures have attempted to address the economic problems of their participants in an era of limited reimbursement, few if any have addressed the concerns of payers. Most such ventures are designed to generate revenues, yet payers aim to reduce expenditures. In order to meet their own objectives, payers have begun to establish negotiated contractual arrangements with both physician and hospital providers. These arrangements vary from simple fee schedules for panels of "preferred" providers to capitated payments and rigorous treatment protocols. In one sense, these contractual arrangements represent the ultimate health care joint venture—among physician, facility, and payer.

Whether these ventures are PPAs or HMOs, they are generally intended to provide payers with mechanisms to control expenditures. Because the control of expenditures requires some control over utilization, these contracts tend to create an adversarial relationship between payer and provider. Coupled with growing competition between physicians and hospitals, the introduction of utilization controls in these ventures has raised new questions about physician-hospital relationships. As a result, many of the long-standing tensions in these relationships have been exacerbated.

A Network Model: Who's the Boss?

When analyzing current changes in the health care system, it is all too easy to focus on the ultimate purchasers and to conclude that, because they control the flow of patients and capital, they can and will control the entire system. Although that conclusion may be essentially correct, to conclude that control will be exercised on a simple economic basis is to assume that health care is a simple economic commodity, not susceptible to variation or to the influences of other constituent parties. In fact, the relationship between physicians and hospitals in a network—be it a PPA, an HMO, or any predetermined package of services—can exert a powerful influence on the system's organization and product.

For the purposes of analysis, let us assume that there are five unrelated parties to a network: a purchaser, an insurer/broker, a group of physicians, a hospital, and patients. The purchaser, who explicitly wants to control the system, will define the desired product. The insurer/broker will work independently with the hospital and the physicians to build the system that will produce it. By working independently with the hospital and physicians, the insurer/broker strengthens the purchaser's negotiating position vis-a-vis each party.* If the insurer/broker wanted to create the strongest negotiating position for the purchaser, network physicians would probably also be drawn from among independent practitioners rather than solely from members of a single organized group practice.

The Role of Relationships

Even in this scenario, which projects an extreme absence of formal relationships among network members, relationships among providers inevitably exist or are formed by creation of the network itself. These, in turn, can play an important role in determining how much and what kind of influence the purchaser develops.

For example, the network physicians in this example are likely to practice geographically close to the network hospital. Thus they have a previously existing relationship with the facility and its medical staff: they are or are not already active admitters to the hospital. If the network physicians are active admitters, active staff members who are not included

---

*In addition, the Wisconsin Attorney General has suggested that, even under current law, if physicians and hospitals work independently with an unrelated broker to create networks or joint ventures, the grounds for antitrust action would be virtually eliminated.[4]

in the network could perceive that the hospital had betrayed them by cooperating with and supporting competitor physicians.

In addition, networks tend to require significant numbers of generalists; therefore, each network physician who is not already on staff may represent not only a potential competitor to the current staff but also a change in the net balance of the staff. Because different types of practices (family practice and orthopedic surgery, for example) create different equipment and staffing requirements, the balance of physicians on staff can be an important factor in determining how the facility's resources are allocated.

These essentially economic factors in medical staff relationships could well cause widespread discontent within the staff and lead to intense physician-to-physician competition. Thus caught between an economically driven medical staff and a purchaser for whom economics is a powerful motive, the hospital would almost inevitably make economic decisions as well. In this scenario, then, the purchaser would indeed exercise control on an economic basis because of the general absence of other countervailing forces.

Beyond Economics

There may, however, be strong forces toward cohesiveness, both among the network physicians and between the network and the rest of the medical staff. If incentives for patients to stay within the network are strong, the network physicians may begin to develop referral patterns among themselves. This interdependence is likely to generate some sense of group identity. If the purchaser has tried to exercise control by imposing stringent treatment protocols or high levels of financial risk on physicians, group identity may also be reinforced in opposition to the purchaser. Even if the underlying motives for this opposition are economic, physicians are not likely to express them in economic terms: the purchaser's strongest claims are economic, and within that paradigm the impositions are appropriate. In order to have an impact, physicians must negate the paradigm.

In their efforts to impose an alternative paradigm, physicians can rely not only on professional expertise and ethics, but also on organizational responsibility. Their "weapon" is quality of care. Particularly if the network physicians can act in concert with the rest of the medical staff, they have a legitimate position from which to exercise that weapon. The law confers upon the organized medical staff of a hospital the responsibility for overseeing and assuring the quality of care delivered by anyone who has clinical privileges in the facility. Thus, caught between two overtly opposing forces, the physicians' demand for quality and the purchasers' demand for cost-effectiveness, the hospital must balance its decisions carefully: it stands to lose revenue if it loses the purchaser, and patients if it loses the doctors who must treat them.

If the whole organized medical staff were willing to support the network physicians (for example, by using its review committees to document the inadequacy of care demanded by a particular utilization-review system), the purchaser would be hard pressed simply to replace dissident network physicians with more economically oriented doctors. Thus, appropriate use of clinical expertise and cohesiveness of physician demands can introduce a noneconomic element into the health care system, even if it is essentially an economic system.

Lessons from the Real World

There is, of course, a large gap between any hypothetical model and reality. In the real world, network relationships are more variable and complex: each organization has more driving forces, each physician has more complex motives, and there is always the possibility of illogical or inconsistent behavior by any of the participating parties.

The previous model was intended, however, only to illustrate two pivotal and related principles that can affect the development of health care systems: the devastating consequences of unfettered economic competition in the health care system, and the importance of the medical staff's independent responsibility for the quality of patient care.

There is currently considerable debate about whether hospital medical staffs have the right to act as independent associations. Some hospitals, feeling pressure from payers and purchasers, argue—or simply choose to behave as though—medical staffs do not have the right to act independently. Physicians increasingly say they do. The arguments involve complex legal reasoning[4] that is beyond the scope of this chapter. However, the two positions may represent extremes that could be modified to the benefit of all parties. It is therefore worth considering the potential impact of each position and the compromises that might contribute to improvements in the future health delivery system.

If the organized medical staff does not have an independent voice, that is, it is completely subsumed under the hospital and its governing board, the health care system may well become a system entirely guided by financial principles.

Hospitals are complex institutions that require significant capital resources to operate. To ensure access to the requisite capital, many hospitals and hospital systems have sought direct relationships with purchasers. Some of these relationships have taken the form of joint ventures (the Voluntary Hospitals of America and Aetna, for example). Others are ventures sponsored by hospitals' own parent companies (such as American Medical International's AMICARE or HealthWest's CareAmerica). In addition, some independent insurers have found it most efficient to contract first with hospitals and then draw network physicians from among the contract hospitals' active medical staffs.

Whatever the structure of these arrangements, they create a strong alliance between hospital and payer, which inevitably creates financial pressures on hospital managers. Moreover, as an increasing number of patients subscribe to these payer-hospital alliances, physicians will themselves be subject to stronger financial pressures than they were under more informal collegial referral relationships.[5]

If hospitals and their medical staffs respond unquestioningly to these economic forces, they may find that they are administering a system of rigidly controlled ''cookbook medicine.'' In such a system, physicians will have abdicated their role as key clinical decision makers in the health care system. There will be little room for them to exercise clinical judgment or creative leadership. Even if the quality of medical practice can be maintained, it will remain at today's levels; the traditional dynamism of the American health care system will be lost. Physicians who seek the intellectual challenge of developing more sophisticated, better documented, and potentially more cost-effective standards of care will find that they are forced to leave mainstream medicine. In the end, health care will have lost the capability of creating exactly the kind of system to which it currently aspires.[6]

An alternative is for health care administrators to recognize the value of their medical staffs and of the physician perspective. There is no question that inviting active physician participation in hospital and network decision-making processes may create some initial difficulties; indeed, no other outcome may be possible if hospitals and physicians regard or use the process as an economic tug-of-war. However, if the parties are motivated to engage in an open discussion of patient care issues, clinical data can be brought to financial decisions and economic realities can become a more integral part of the clinical process. Only when the boundaries between administration and clinical care become permeable in this way will it be possible to contemplate what compromises can—much less, should—be made in support of patient care.

Ultimately, the guiding principles of medical staff relations in health care networks may force the entire system to examine the purpose it serves. If it is to be nothing more than an ongoing system for allocating health care resources, then the competitive economic model may be appropriate. In this model, it would be entirely appropriate to deal with physicians as if they were simply technically skilled workers. If, however, the overall goal of the American health care system is to provide high-quality, comprehensive patient care—even in a cost-effective manner—the professional expertise of physicians can only be a valuable addition to any hospital's planning or decision-making process.

References

1. American Medical Association, Board of Trustees. *Integration of the Health Care Sector: Definitions, Trends, and Implication.* Report GG, I-85. Chicago: AMA, 1985.

2. Starr, P. *The Social Transformation of American Medicine.* New York: Basic Books, 1982.
3. Richman, D. Federal investigations scrutinizing hospitals' physician incentive plans. *Modern Healthcare.* 1985, Oct. 25. 15(22):24.
4. American Medical Association, Board of Trustees. *Hospital-Medical Staff Joint Ventures: An Update.* Report Q, I-85. Chicago: AMA, 1985.
5. Willett, D. E. *What Physicians Should Know About the Legal Status of the Medical Staff.* San Francisco: California Medical Association, 1984.
6. Wolinsky, F. D., and Marder, W. D. *The Organization of Medical Practice and the Practice of Medicine,* Ann Arbor, MI: Health Administrative Press, 1985, *passim.*
7. Bridgeman, J. F. Balkanization of a proud profession. *The California Internist.* Fall, 1985. 40(3): 2.

Chapter 5

Strategies for Hospital-Physician Cooperation

Steven W. Lewis, M.D.

Many are predicting that the days of the stand-alone hospital are numbered. Experts disagree as to how long such institutions can survive, but many are giving them less than a few years. Gradually replacing the stand-alone facility are provider systems that span the service spectrum from small, rural, primary care facilities to sophisticated tertiary care centers. Such networks will form more frequently over the next several years.

Simple networking of unrelated facilities is not enough, however, to survive current economic pressures. The real survivors will be those who go beyond the simple acquisition of multiple hospitals to true horizontal integration of services and facilities and creation of a comprehensive continuum of care. This is happening already in both investor-owned and not-for-profit sectors.

In addition to horizontal integration, networked systems are moving in the direction of managed health care. Managed plans, which try to secure a patient base through integration of a finance mechanism and delivery system, constitute what is called *vertical integration.* Current economic forces are therefore creating significant pressures for the development of comprehensive delivery systems integrated with financing systems. These structural changes, in turn, are bringing about changes in traditional hospital-physician relations. The old rules governing these relations can, in fact, be very counterproductive in this new era.

If physicians and integrated delivery systems are to work together productively, a new relationship is required. It must be flexible enough to accommodate various market segments and a rapidly changing environment. Yet it must be predictable enough so that managed care systems can offer uniformly cost-effective care and, thereby, compete.

Traditional Hospital-Physician Relations

In general, hospital-physician relations were successful in the past. Although the cost of care grew to excessive proportions and access to care was not ideal

Dr. Lewis is Vice-President for Medical Affairs, Intermountain Health Care, Inc., Salt Lake City, UT.

for all, on the whole the relationship worked reasonably well. Certainly, most physicians have been pleased with both the economic and the professional rewards that the practice of medicine offered over the past 20 years.

Hospitals, too, were rewarded for the contribution they made to the well-being of their communities. There seemed to be an endless stream of dollars for health care, and the only pressures that existed were largely those of expanding services appropriately and ensuring that high-quality care was the outcome. Physician involvement with hospitals came about largely through the medical staff. Physicians also held positions on governing boards and were often invited to participate in planning. In the main, however, the economic interests of hospitals and physicians were intertwined because of their mutual involvement in the delivery of care. There were few formal channels of joint decision making. There was almost no joint risk taking, except in some joint ventures.

Despite the lack of formalized joint decision making, hospitals and physicians did, over time, have an increasing economic impact on one another. Tension would mount, for example, between physicians affected positively and those affected negatively by a hospital action. Occasionally, a whole staff would be involved in an issue of economic or other importance, and then relations in general would be strained. Once a solution was reached physicians and hospitals would resume their old ways. Both parties would essentially go their own way, getting along most of the time because of generally good times for the health care industry as a whole. Thus, there were few consistent pressures on the relationship.

The key interface between the hospital and the medical staff was the hospital administrator. When problems arose, the administrator managed the solution from the hospital's perspective. Interaction with physicians was focused at the administrator level, even in most larger systems. There was no ''corporate'' relationship then.

As economic change forced hospitals to network, to enter the managed health care arena, and to make themselves efficient enough to be viable in a prospective payment era, they soon found that the very nature of hospital-physician relations hindered their efforts. The traditional administrator-based, one-to-one-style relationship with physicians prevented hospitals from responding quickly and meaningfully to the changes in the marketplace. To understand why, it is necessary to examine some of the issues brought about by the new economic environment that are affecting hospital-physician relations.

Toward a New Relationship: Issues Both Parties Must Resolve

The switch to risk-sharing prospective payment systems increased requirements for cost efficiency in the delivery of care, and the need for more cost-effective physician practice styles have prompted hospitals to seek better relationships with physicians. Physicians, likewise, are motivated to seek better relationships with hospitals and hospital corporations in order to ensure patient access and, thus, a stable economic future for themselves.

Solo practitioners and physicians in small groups feel vulnerable and unable to adequately respond to demands being placed on them by payers. Looking for viable partners, these physicians recognize that hospitals and systems may be able to provide the edge they need to guarantee secure practices. There is a small problem of trust, however. There is also the question of control.

The Issue of Trust

Trust, or having confidence in one another's motives, was not a vital ingredient for productive hospital-physician relations in the past. There was little need for it to develop, because both parties were fairly autonomous. The few exceptions were those instances where a hospital action directly affected physicians, such as building an urgent care center that competed with primary care physicians for patients.

Today, trust is the foundation upon which effective competitive partnerships are built. It is vital to moving ahead. It must be given time to evolve, but it must also be encouraged and worked on by all involved parties. Trust will develop as both hospitals and physicians move toward the businesslike style of interaction necessary to achieve a sustained, competitive edge. The key is for both parties to agree on goals that establish mutually beneficial financial incentives (see Long-Term Objectives, p. 48, for more information).

The Issue of Control

Physicians feel they have lost control of the health care delivery system and are being acted upon without being involved in the decision making. On the other hand, hospitals, and especially hospital systems, are asking, "What do physicians bring to the table such that we should relinquish control to them?"

Both sides raise legitimate concerns. Physicians cannot expect to participate with parity, for example, in the capital decision-making processes of a multimillion dollar system, when they have no risk in the decisions made. Likewise, hospitals cannot assume that physicians, who are among the most independent of professionals, will suddenly fall in line and begin behaving as hospital managers wish, unless they are appropriately involved in decision making.

The solution is to involve physicians in decision making, as appropriate. Physicians can make valuable contributions to many hospital decisions. Hospital managers who realize that fact will enjoy an advantage over those who have not learned to effectively include physicians. Some decisions will involve physicians more than others, especially issues that have a direct impact on clinical medicine. Sometimes, physicians will need help in understanding cost and other constraints on delivery styles, but decisions as to what makes sense clinically should be left largely to them.

Much has been written about the control issue. Most writers conclude that control decisions should be based on what makes the most sense in the marketplace. Thus, over time, hospitals and physicians will work out what makes the most sense in a given situation.

Long-Term Objectives

As the issues of trust and control are being negotiated, the two parties must come to some agreement on long-term objectives. Following are some important objectives to consider:

- *Economic security.* This is clearly a goal of both physicians and hospitals. To achieve it, they must demonstrate an ability to compete under the new rules of a price-sensitive marketplace. Active involvement in managed care systems will contribute to economic security by providing hospitals and physicians with ready access to patient groups.
- *Physician representation in the hospital decision-making process.* This should, of course, be a physician goal. But responsible physician input into and support of hospital policy will also rebound to the competitive advantage of hospitals. In order to be involved in decision making, each physician will have to give up the notion that no one can represent his views. Administrators will need to continue to provide one-on-one "high-touch" interactions with physicians, however, so that each physician will feel that his opinion is valued.
- *A high level of predictability.* Both hospitals and physicians require this of each other. Hospitals need a high degree of predictability in physician relations, if they are to enter the managed care market and succeed. To compete effectively, managed care plans must be cost-efficient. The only way to guarantee long-term cost-effectiveness is to follow efficient utilization patterns. Hospitals therefore need a predictable commitment to efficient utilization from their physician partners. Equally essential is predictably high-quality care.

    Physicians, too, require predictability in their new partners in health care delivery and financing. They need to count on having a consistent voice in determining the principles of risk assumption that will structure a health care plan. They must also be assured of consistently having input into determining acceptable

patterns of clinical practice in a plan.
- *Congruence of financial incentives.* This is another essential component of a solid partnership between hospitals and physicians. If both parties are confident that they will benefit financially in ways that are mutually productive, trust will soar. But, in some ways, hospitals and physicians will be in competition, especially as the world of outpatient medicine expands. Insofar as possible, both parties must agree that mutually beneficial actions will have priority. Areas of potential competition must also be discussed, and, together, physicians and administration should determine how to deal with them. Creation of this congruence will be difficult and the nature of it will vary from place to place, but it is a key to successful hospital-physician relations.

If hospitals and physicians deal with all these issues and objectives successfully, chances are that mutual loyalty will result. Loyalty means that, given reasonable options, the parties will choose to do that which is mutually productive, at least on the average. Once loyalty has been achieved, and it never will be completely, the two parties will have attained a ''partner-like'' relationship.

What Both Parties Bring to the Partnership

Both physicians and hospitals bring much to the partnership table: hospitals, their financial, marketing, and management strengths; physicians, their expertise in the clinical delivery area and access to patients through traditional lines of referral.

Hospitals, and systems in particular, increasingly will control access to patient flow. Their entry into managed health care will provide a large portion of this control. In addition, hospital contracts to deliver services to other plans and major health care purchasers will further increase access to patients. The importance of these avenues of access to physicians will be more crucial as time goes on.

The marketing and management expertise that hospitals typically possess will also be critical elements of success in the future. Top management skills will be required as hospitals themselves seek more efficient ways of providing the same levels of care. Physicians will also need managerial know-how to keep operational costs in line as increasing patient volume becomes a less reliable means of maintaining income. In addition, marketing skills must be developed if physicians, and hospitals, are to retain their competitive advantage.

Physicians, on the other hand, direct the delivery of care. They are experts in the caring and curing functions. What this means in a competitive marketplace is that physicians, with the proper incentives, should know how, or be able to determine how, to deliver high-quality care very efficiently. Physicians are also in the best position to understand what patients really want. Thus, they can be real allies in marketing.

Physicians' expertise is also necessary in the technology review process, as well as determining how best to use the new technology. Moreover, physicians can provide valuable input when hospitals consider new managed care products, new services, and new vehicles of access that will attract more patients to a managed care system. In short, there is much to be gained from a partnership between physicians and hospitals/systems, as long as each side recognizes that the other has a legitimate claim to having a strong position.

Forging the New Partnership

The concept of partnership is laudable and seems a worthy goal. But how, in this new, tough, competitive, and not all that forgiving world of health care delivery and financing, do hospitals and physicians go about creating a durable partnership?

Avoid Quick Fixes

One key is to *avoid quick fixes*. Short-term solutions that create adverse long-term incentives with resultant lack of marketplace responsiveness are worse than doing nothing at all. A finger-in-the-dike approach may be needed in a few situations, but to engage in "sufficing activities" as standard practice is shortsighted and, in the long term, counterproductive.

An example of such a quick fix is to put together a joint venture and wait for hospital-physician-relationship problems to disappear. However, instead of disappearing, the problems are likely to increase. Worse yet, a managed care system that is launched before laying the proper groundwork with physicians could turn into the worst possible nightmare, with little chance of success.

It is important to understand that none of the many possible ventures or corporate setups being advanced today are in and of themselves long-term cures for physician relationship problems. The basic ingredients of good hospital-physician relations must already be in place or at least under development before launching a joint venture. At best, the planning phase of a new venture can help cement an already good relationship.

Establish an Open Dialogue

The best way to start building a good relationship is carefully and openly. The process chosen to work out an improved, tighter, more responsible, and responsive relationship will in large part determine its success. There are many approaches that can be taken. Hospitals can draw up a management "bill of rights" on which they will not negotiate. Physicians can define turf from which they will not budge. In some cases, this approach may be necessary. However, it always makes a compromise solution more difficult to achieve.

The sooner open dialogue can begin, the better. Physicians must be made aware of hospital industry changes. Hospitals must develop a better and more in-depth understanding of the realities of the private practice of medicine. Mutual fears must be shared. Appropriate history must come to light, so each side can better understand the other's perspective. So far, no plans or hard issues have been discussed. This is all just simple human relations, characterized by an adult, businesslike interaction.

Once the concerns, strengths, and fears of both sides have had an adequate airing (adequate, but not exhaustive), the parties should formulate a plan of action. Again, this should be an open process. All who can and want to be involved insofar as makes competitive sense, should be involved. The risk of this approach is that not all will have an equal understanding or equal abilities, and certainly not all will be in agreement with any given direction. However, consensus is not the purpose. Openness is. Openness will ensure not only fairness, but also better results.

An open approach also allows for self-selection to occur. Not all physicians will want to be involved. Some will opt out early, maybe angrily, but they will have left voluntarily. Self-selection thus lays the groundwork for a tighter relationship with those physicians who decide to stay involved. To close the doors instead, make decisions with a select friendly few, and then try to sell the product to all physicians is an uphill battle. The open method develops physician and administrative champions who sell the program or venture willingly and with a higher probability of success.

Minimize Change

Common sense also dictates that the creation of a physician relationship responsive to the current marketplace must be done with as little disruption of past ways as possible. Economic change has already rocked the professional culture of the private practitioner and has had a significant impact on the hospital as well. To enter into a relationship with physicians that brings unnecessary further change will only result in disaster. Thus, a major goal in the early planning and decision-making stages is to determine those areas where change is necessary, and those where change should not occur.

In general, there are two areas where change will need to occur. One requires significant change on the part of physicians, and one on the part of hospitals.

The nature of the economic relationship between hospitals and physicians will bring with it dramatic change for physicians. Managed health care, for example, entails fee schedules, financial risk-sharing, and modification of practice styles. The cultural impact on physicians because of these basic economic changes is marked. Hospitals should therefore buffer that impact as much as reasonably possible. One effective way is to involve physicians in the structuring of risk-sharing principles.

Hospitals, on their part, undergo significant cultural shock as they involve physicians in policy making and governance. Direct involvement in management brings with it an even more profound impact. Hospitals risk dramatic change in the usual mechanisms of decision making, not to mention the outcome of the decision-making process.

To lessen the impact, physicians must assume some risk for the decisions they help make. The proper physician organization will help, but only if the necessary groundwork has been laid. (See chapter 1 for a discussion of various organizational models.) However, it is important to note that imposing the model or structure does not make the organization. For example, if a physician organization were put together that was not truly built on principles of physician representation[1] then any decision made by that body would meet with resistance. Simply having the organization is not sufficient to satisfy relationship needs.

Future Challenges

The marketplace will be the shaping force of the future, and the survivors will be those who carefully track and proactively respond to it. But, for those who are not trendsetters, there will always be market niches that will provide a viable future. Whether trendsetters or followers, the winners will be those who are in tune with the market.

New skills never before needed in the health care field will become more and more necessary. Marketing, advertising, packaging, and selling are already important skills and will become even more so in the future. Services will expand, effective marketing to promote them will be required, and the spectrum of financing mechanisms necessary to deal with payers will broaden. All of these trends will place stress on hospital-physician relations.

Increasingly, hospitals will have to deal with the tension between having "adequate" physician involvement in new initiatives and being flexible and quick enough to respond to market changes. Winning players, be they physicians or hospitals, will find that they must tie themselves more closely to their health care delivery counterparts.

This closeness will be in the form of increased mutual risk-sharing. In the price-sensitive managed care arena, how a premium is developed, split, and distributed will become an issue of mutual concern and decision making. Hospitals will find that their participation in networked systems leads to the regionalization of services. They will strengthen some services, but give up others, so that the system as a whole can be more cost-effective and competitive. This, in turn, will have dramatic implications for their medical staffs. More and more destinies will become intertwined. More and more relationships will become closer. More and more, the winners will behave in a mutually beneficial way.

The most difficult of future tasks, however, will be to accomplish all this in the absence of total, or even near-total, congruence of interests. For example, although the fee-for-service world will shrink dramatically and the managed care world will grow, physicians and hospitals will find it necessary to operate in both worlds. At times, this will seemingly put them at odds with each other; at times this will seemingly put them at odds with themselves.

The winners will negotiate the difficulties of a world changing from fee-for-service and cost reimbursement to one of cost containment and managed delivery of care without losing their balanced approach. There is no formula that hospitals and physicians can use to predict the proper balance. But it is vital that whatever the approach taken, both parties agree upon it. Such open agreement and decision making spreads the risk. Otherwise, one side will always find reason to blame the other for untoward outcomes of a joint decision.

The future includes these known challenges, as well as several unknowns. The hospitals and systems that will prove successful will be those who, among other right moves, work out a close and flexible relationship with physicians.

Summary

Horizontal and vertical integration of hospitals and hospital systems will continue to be the direction of progressive health care delivery players for the immediate future. Entry into the managed health care arena will be a major result of these integration efforts. Not only will these trends impose new stresses on hospital-physician relationships, but effective responses to them will be impossible unless hospitals establish new and closer ties with physicians.

Hospitals will choose their new partners indirectly, by offering to engage physicians actively in decision making, governance, and financial risk-sharing, and by developing a greater mutuality of interests with them. Uninterested physicians will pass up the offers. Others will become involved to a limited extent, as a way of hedging their bets. Still others will participate fully and win as their partner wins.

The prospect of closer hospital-physician relations brings with it some major challenges. But, more important, it offers a significant opportunity for new, mutual successes.

Reference

1. Shortell, S. M., and others. The medical staff of the future: Replanting the garden. *Frontiers of Health Services Management. 1985 Feb. 1(3):3-48.*

Chapter 6

How to Pay Doctors: Implications of Trends and Available Data

Stephen F. Jencks, M.D.

Paying physicians is an expensive, controversial, and sensitive process. Medicare, as well as other insurers, is exploring possible changes in payment methods. Many proposals center on bundling individual services or hospital admissions, or going the capitation route. Some of the controversy surrounding payment method can be reduced, or at least tempered, by familiarity with recent trends and findings. The most important conclusion to be drawn from these findings is that competition may be a more effective strategy than additional regulatory rate-setting in reducing costs for Medicare and other insurers.

Although reform of Medicare's physician payment process has many goals, they can be summarized as follows: Through a combination of incentives for efficiency and competitive price setting, control the growth of governmental and beneficiary liability while maintaining access to quality care.

Payment Trends

Medicare's current interest in physician payments springs primarily from the extraordinary growth in outlays for physician services. From 1980 to 1983, outlays for Medicare's Part B program grew 20 percent a year—even more rapidly than payments to hospitals. But at the end of 1984, the rate of increase dropped to about 6 percent a year. This drop resulted in part from the freeze legislated in June 1984 but also from a longer-term trend, which began to emerge in 1983, about the time Medicare's hospital Prospective Payment System (PPS) was implemented. The longer-term trend may be due not only to PPS, but to concurrent private-sector pressures, and other forces.

Available Treasury data indicate that physicians have not substantially increased volume or intensity of services in response to the freeze, although

Dr. Jencks is Research Physician, Health Care Financing Administration, Baltimore, MD.

The research reported in this chapter was current as of July 1985.

other data on this question are still being analyzed. The decreased growth
rate may therefore reduce pressure for physician payment reform in the
short run. But the decline provides no clues as to what Medicare should do
after the freeze.

Assignment Rates

A physician who accepts assignment on a Medicare bill agrees to Medicare's
determination of the allowable charge as payment in full for service. On
average, the allowable charge is 25 percent less than the physician's billed
charge (Health Care Financing Administration, unpublished data).

A key to controlling the growth of beneficiary liability is an increase in
physician assignment rates. Physician refusal of assignment is a special
problem because almost no "Medigap" policies cover this component of
costs. As a remedy, some policymakers have suggested mandatory assignment for all physician services.

From 1976 to 1983, the rate of acceptance of assignment rose very
gradually from 50 percent of claims to 54 percent of claims. But from 1984 to
mid-1985, the rate rose very rapidly to almost 70 percent of claims and 65
percent of dollars, and is still rising (HCFA, unpublished data). This increase
has been accelerated both by mandatory assignment of independent laboratory bills and by Medicare's Participating Physician (MPP) Program, but is
substantial even after those factors are considered. In light of this rapid and
continuing rise, arguments for mandatory assignment have lost much of
their force. The rising assignment trend remains, however, extremely uneven:
while the average rate is 69.4 percent, it is under 40 percent in the Dakotas
and above 90 percent in Massachusetts and Rhode Island.

The MPP program, legislated in 1984, was successful in enrolling
almost a third of physicians who see Medicare beneficiaries; these physicians account for more than a third of all beneficiary services. This is
impressive for a program that was promoted for only a few months before
the sign-up period ended and was not fully understood by many physicians.
Nevertheless, enrollment was almost as uneven across states as the rate of
acceptance of assignment. Possible enhancements to make the MPP program more attractive might include even greater publicity, making billing
easier, and increasing distribution of MPP lists to providers and beneficiaries.

Impact of Competitive Pressures

Competitive pressures have contributed to increasing acceptance of assignment and can be expected to push more physicians toward becoming MPPs.
Pressures, such as the increased physician supply, Medicare's PPS, private-
sector cost containment, and the growth of health maintenance organizations (HMOs), will also make physician payment reform easier and perhaps

inevitable. The absence of such a competitive response over the past 20 years, as the physician supply has grown, led many economists and planners to believe that producing more physicians would only increase health care costs. However, physicians are now locating in areas where they would never have located in the past, accepting entry-level pay that they would never have accepted, offering discounts to insurers and preferred provider systems, and experiencing very real pressure on their incomes.[1]

A recent Gallup poll reported that 12 percent of physicians have actually reduced fees in response to competition from HMOs.[2] Other evidence suggests that consumer resistance has combined with the growing physician supply to end physicians' general ability to increase fees and service volume. For example, primary care physicians should be able to generate demand more easily than other specialists; however, primary care incomes have fallen.[3] Perhaps the most dramatic single example of consumer resistance to rising physician payments is the Medicare physician payment freeze enacted in 1984. Although the results of the freeze are still being analyzed, it appears that if purchasers such as Medicare use competition to bargain for lower prices, increased physician supply may actually lower total costs.

The Health Insurance Revolution

In the past few years, the whole health insurance market has been revolutionized. Insurers who defined their job as paying bills expeditiously found themselves losing market share to insurers who promised to contain health care costs. As a result, many insurers have become increasingly involved in providing health care services:

- Insurers have launched their own HMOs. HMOs merge the function of providing services with the insuring function in a single organization.
- Insurance companies have been acquired by hospital systems.
- Insurers have increasingly screened for the necessity for admissions, have included service location as part of the definition of benefits, and have redefined the package of services for which payment will be made.
- Insurers have negotiated directly with providers regarding charges and discounts.

Not all insurers have adopted the same strategy. While Medicare is putting pressure on hospitals to reduce cost per admission, commercial insurers and Blue Cross/Blue Shield seem to be concentrating on averting admissions through screening and ambulatory surgery. These two approaches have apparently had a synergistic effect, resulting in decreased costs per admission in the nonfederal sector and decreased Medicare admissions.

Constant dollar payments for inpatient services actually fell for the majority of Blue Cross plans in 1984 (Blue Cross Association, unpublished data). Such synergy appears desirable in physician services as well.

Regional Variations

As noted earlier, acceptance of assignment and enrollment in the MPP program vary widely. In addition, although physician incomes have fallen in some parts of the country, they have forged ahead of inflation in others. Competition is established and intense in some regions, but only beginning to be felt in others. Such diversity suggests that many problems are local and require local, rather than national, solutions and that when solutions are national in scope they should be extremely flexible.

Payment Reform: Three Bundling Options

A major feature of Medicare hospital reimbursement policy is the aggregation of services into larger payment units, or "bundling." Three levels of bundling have been proposed for physician payment:

- The individual service (current fee for service).
- The hospital admission (payment of a single sum for all physician services during an admission, using DRGs).
- One year of service (pay a single sum for all covered physician services during the year, using capitation).

As the bundle becomes larger, controlling volume becomes easier, but paying accurately for the bundle becomes more difficult. Nevertheless, bundling is an effective tool for cost containment because it encourages efficiency and reduces the incentive to produce more individual services or to provide individual services of greater complexity and cost. Evidence that physicians are now more constrained in increasing services suggests, however, that bundling may be less critical to controlling physician costs than hospital costs. In addition, bundled hospital services appear to have had secondary effects on certain kinds of physician services, such as radiology.

The Individual Service Approach

Medicare now sets physician payments using the customary (the physician's customary submitted charge), prevailing (the prevailing submitted charge in the community), and reasonable (a criterion usually applied when charge data is unavailable)—CPR—system. Currently, the CPR system has few supporters because:

- Its complexity prevents beneficiaries from easily predicting what Medicare will pay.
- Prices seem to vary among physicians and geographic areas in ways that are difficult to explain.
- It encourages charges to rise and puts no pressure on them to fall back, even if underlying costs fall.
- It provides greater profit for performing procedures (with high overhead), rather than more routine services, such as physical examinations and careful history-taking. It also encourages the introduction of expensive new procedures.
- It assumes that physicians customarily receive their posted charges, when discounting is actually widespread.
- It encourages specialization and location in areas of physician oversupply.

Almost all other countries with some form of government-sponsored health insurance use more direct ways of setting payments than CPR and do not rely on submitted charges.[4] The usual approach is a fee schedule based on a relative value scale (RVS). An RVS is a table of weights that define relative prices for procedures; a conversion factor or multiplier converts the relative value into a dollar price. RVSs are derived from varying combinations of historical prices, theoretical studies, and professional consensus. In other countries, RVSs tend to be under the control of organized medicine, and the factors used to convert relative values into actual payments are determined by insurers or the government.

If HCFA wished to implement the RVS concept in the United States, it might use a three-stage strategy:

- Develop fee schedules based on current charges or payments.
- Adjust fees for procedures that appear to be over- or under-priced.
- Base payments increasingly on RVSs, which would become increasingly national in scope.

Drawbacks

But there are some potential drawbacks to using RVSs:

- It is not clear how much consensus regarding relative values exists now or could be developed between consumers, providers, and Medicare.
- RVSs do not prevent increases in the volume and intensity of services, and payment controls have historically resulted in increased volume and intensity of service.[5,6] There is some evidence that physicians can no longer initiate increases in order to

achieve target incomes, and Medicare might adjust payments downward if unexpected increases in volume took place.

- Evidence of regional variations, especially in the supply of certain specialties, suggests that national strategies may be much less effective in seeking to drive down Medicare costs through competition. Strategies might result in competitive prices in the average community but in overpayments or access barriers in others.
- The Federal Trade Commission (FTC) expressed specific concerns regarding the anticompetitive impact of RVSs in an advisory letter to the American Society of Internal Medicine.[7] Those concerns focused on two major issues: (1) the probability that an RVS would be slanted by its developers to increase the income of particular groups, and (2) the likelihood that an RVS would primarily be a tool for price-setting by buyers, rather than payment negotiation by payers. The use of national scales by HCFA, where HCFA would be determining total payments, would not appear to raise either of these dangers.

The Access Issue

A critical consideration in reforming physician payment is the impact on Medicare beneficiaries' access to care. Several kinds of data bear on this issue. First, there is no evidence that the current Medicare fee freeze has reduced Medicare beneficiaries' access to care. Nor is there evidence that many beneficiaries are unable to secure care because Medicare's current payments are too low. Second, available data suggest that although payments for certain technically based procedures may be too high, payments for more cognitively oriented procedures are not demonstrably too low. Finally, the fact that physician acceptance of assignment continued to increase in the midst of the freeze suggests competitive pressures that could allow lower payments for individual physician services without decreased access.

Medicare's goal is to pay just enough to ensure continued access to good care for Medicare beneficiaries. It is possible within the Medicare system to monitor access to care through a fairly simple strategy. Under this strategy, Medicare would continuously monitor the degree to which service delivery is concentrated in just a few physicians. If Medicare beneficiaries are securing care from as many physicians after a change in payment as before, one could conclude that the change has not impaired access to care. Comparisons with the number of physicians serving beneficiaries in other health insurance programs would provide further information on access.

The DRG Approach

The key policy issues in the DRG approach are how much to pay, what to pay for, whom to pay, and whether the strategy is advisable.

How Much to Pay

Extensive empirical work indicates that, when payments are aggregated at the hospital or medical staff level, DRGs predict current Medicare physician payments for an admission even better than they predicted pre-PPS payments to hospitals.[8,9] However, DRGs do not perform equally well for all classes of admissions. They are good predictors for surgical cases (for both physician and hospital payments), but poor for nonsurgical cases (for both kinds of payments). Thus, DRGs would be an adequate tool for determining how much to pay at the hospital or medical staff level, but not at the individual physician level if nonsurgeons were included.

What to Pay For

One empirical question is whether preadmission or postdischarge care should be included in a DRG-based payment. Research has not revealed any particular length of time for which such services should be included, but they do not currently represent a large fraction of inpatient physician payments.[9] The limitation of the empirical data is that it does not predict changes in service patterns that might result from implementing a DRG-based physician payment system.

A second question, whether all physician services should be included in such a payment, is addressed in the forthcoming section, ''Advisability of the DRG Approach.''

Whom to Pay

Because the DRG system does not work well for nonsurgical cases, it is not feasible to use it for paying individual physicians. If a DRG-type system were used to pay at the medical staff level, the problem of acceptance of assignment would be important. If the medical staff or hospital were free to accept or refuse assignment on a case-by-case basis, potential beneficiary liability would rise significantly upon transition to a DRG-based system.

In a DRG-based system, Medicare would make a DRG-based average payment for each hospitalization assigned to a particular DRG, regardless of the physician services provided to the particular patient. If assignment were accepted for low-cost cases and refused for high-cost cases, beneficiary liability for high-cost cases would be substantially greater than under the present system. Beneficiaries would become liable for the difference between the high charges in their case and the Medicare payment. Liability would also rise for low-cost cases if coinsurance were defined as 20 percent of Medicare's DRG-based payment rather than 20 percent of the bills the physicians would have submitted.

Advisability of the DRG Approach

Solutions to the problems outlined above are complex and may require demonstrations if the DRG approach is to be considered for national implementation. But further data sheds light on the advisability of implementing a DRG strategy for physician payment:

- Data from the past two years indicate that overall growth in inpatient physician costs has moderated dramatically and that noninpatient sectors, instead, have become the primary focus of growth (HCFA, unpublished data). However, there is no ambulatory services classification system that appears adequate for determining physician payments on a DRG-type basis.
- Examination of the composition of inpatient physician payments indicates that the majority are made for surgical and anesthesia charges (HCFA, unpublished data). Because these services are central to the admissions in which they occur, paying by the admission is not likely to reduce the surgery/anesthesia component of cost. Controlling payments for individual services may therefore be a more effective strategy than bundling.

The Capitation Approach

Capitation* appears to be an effective way to save on both physician and hospital payments. Whereas savings on hospital costs in capitated systems result from decreased utilization, savings on physician costs probably result from negotiation of fees or salaries between the capitated entity and the physician and from substitution of nonphysician providers for physicians.

How Much to Pay

There are unresolved problems with respect to Medicare's determination of capitated payments to such entities as HMOs and competitive medical plans. The pricing method, adjusted average per capita cost (AAPCC), may not take complete account of the fact that Medicare beneficiaries enrolling in capitated plans tend to be healthier than those who do not enroll.[10] Although enrollees appear to become more like nonenrollees over time, the problem of enrollment bias remains.

How to Enroll More Beneficiaries

HMOs are growing very rapidly (22 percent enrollment growth in 1984)

---

*Capitation is not limited to HMOs. Capitated payments can also be negotiated under fee-for-service arrangements, such as independent practice associations (IPAs) and other competitive medical plans.

and the annual rate of growth is accelerating quickly (from 10 percent in 1982 to 15 percent in 1983 and 22 percent in 1984). But it is not yet clear whether new regulations will succeed in encouraging large-scale enrollment of Medicare beneficiaries in capitated systems.

Two strategies for increasing the rate of enrollment are vouchers and geographic capitation. *Voucher* is a generic term for strategies under which insurers and other groups could receive the capitated payments, which are currently made only to health care delivery systems. This strategy would enlarge the number of entities that could receive capitated payments, thus accelerating enrollment. *Geographic capitation* describes a system in which insurance-type entities would receive payment on a capitated basis for all Medicare beneficiaries in a geographic area and then be responsible for insuring their care. Current proposals protect against possible anticompetitive features of geographic capitation through the continued availability of traditional Medicare and alternatives such as HMOs and CMPs. Both of these mechanisms have great appeal, but to date there is little empirical evidence regarding either.

Conclusion

The evidence suggests that Medicare and other insurers are entering a period in which effective strategies will need to be extremely flexible. Strategies must respond differently to situations where there is aggressive competition and situations where competition has not made strong inroads. Further data collection and interpretation will be critical for guiding policy and ensuring that payment controls respect Medicare's fiscal responsibility to taxpayers and beneficiaries, as well as for guaranteeing continued access to high-quality medical care.

References

1. Jencks, S., and Dobson, A. Strategies for reforming Medicare's physician payments: physician diagnosis-related groups and other approaches. *New England Journal of Medicine*. 1985. 312(23):1492-1499.
2. Courting MDs for HMOs. *Medical World News*. 1985. 26(12):11-14.
3. American Medical Association. *Average Physician Professional Expenses* and *Net Income after Expenses before Taxes—1983*. SMS Report. 1984 Aug. 3(5):1-4.
4. Reinhardt, U.E. The Compensation of Physicians: Approaches Used in Other Countries. Final report of HCFA Grant 95-P-97309/2. Princeton, NJ: Princeton University, 1985.
5. Rice, T., and McCall, N. Changes in Medicare reimbursement in Colorado: Impact on physicians' economic behavior. *Health Care Financing Review*. 1982. 3(4):67-86.
6. Holohan, J., Scanlon, W., and others. The Effect of Medicare/Medicaid reimbursement on physician behavior. In: Gabel, J. and others, editors. *Physicians and*

Economic Incentives. HCFA Pub 03067. Washington, DC: Health Care Financing Administration, 1980, pp. 43-54.

7. Federal Trade Commission. Advisory opinion to the American Society of Internal Medicine on the legality under the antitrust laws of its relative value guide proposal. Washington, DC: FTC, April 19, 1985.

8. Mitchell, J.B., Calore, K.A., and others. *Physician DRGs: What Do They Look Like and How Would They Work?* Chestnut Hill, MA: Center for Health Economics Research, Feb. 25, 1985.

9. West, H., Marcus, L., and others. Physician and Hospital Reimbursement Study. Report on HHS Contract 100-83-0026. Vienna, VA: Mandex, Inc., Jan. 31, 1985.

10. Eggers, P.W., and Prihoda, R. Pre-enrollment reimbursement patterns of Medicare beneficiaries enrolled in ''at-risk'' HMOs. *Health Care Financing Review.* 1982. 4(1):55-73.

11. Interstudy. National HMO Census, June 30, 1983. Excelsior, MN: Interstudy, 1984.

Chapter 7

Preventing Malpractice Losses: Strategies for Hospital Medical Staffs

William F. Jessee, M.D.

Spiraling medical malpractice losses and insurance premiums have become a major issue in health care. However, providers should avoid a simplistic view of this complex issue. Taking the position that doctors and hospitals are innocent victims of external forces over which they have no control tends to discredit the industry's concern and contribute nothing to resolving the problem.

Indeed, the growth of medical malpractice in the United States is a complex phenomenon that involves social values, changes in the law, increased technological sophistication of medical practice, greater specialization in medical care, and unrealistic public expectations of the benefits of health care. Many of these forces are clearly outside the control of hospitals and physicians. However, physicians and other health professionals are the *only* individuals who can control at least one critical component of the malpractice problem: the quality of care they provide.

Scope of the Problem

The extent of the professional liability problem is well documented. Between 1979 and 1983, the frequency of malpractice claims reported by 23 physician-owned insurance companies more than doubled.[1] In some states, physicians experienced an increase in claims frequency of several hundred percent. For example, the frequency of claims rose in Michigan by 229 percent and in Mississippi by 2,400 percent between 1979 and 1983.[1] Urban areas of the nation, in particular, have experienced a rapid rise in claims.

Assertions by the American Trial Lawyers Association that there has been no real increase in claims frequency and that the purported increase is simply a reflection of larger numbers of health care encounters are not

Dr. Jessee is currently Vice-President of Education, Joint Commission on Accreditation of Hospitals, Chicago. During the development of this chapter, he was Associate Professor, Department of Health Policy and Administration, University of North Carolina School of Public Health, Chapel Hill, NC.

supported by the evidence. In fact, malpractice claims have risen during a period of continually declining hospital census and a relatively stable number of physician-patient encounters.

In addition to the growing frequency of claims, average losses paid per claim rose a hefty 50 percent per year from 1979 to 1985.[1] This figure is climbing partly due to inflation and partly because of an increase in the severity of claims. Of the claims that go to trial, most are still being settled for the defense, favoring the health care industry. However, those decided in favor of the plaintiff are bringing larger and larger awards.

In 1982, the average jury verdict approached $1 million.[1] Neonatal injuries, in particular, have been associated with large verdicts, due in part to the expense of lifelong care. In the wake of these large settlements and judgments, many of the physician-owned mutual professional liability insurance companies, started in the late 70s in response to the "crisis of 1975," have verged on bankruptcy and, in some cases, gone into receivership.

Seeking Solutions

Tort reforms figure prominently in the attempt to ameliorate the rapid rise in the volume and cost of malpractice losses. Current initiatives would:

- Eliminate joint and several liability and collateral source rules
- Cap awards for pain and suffering damages
- Provide for pretrial evaluation by an impartial physician panel, with the evidence presented and conclusions reached available for introduction at trial
- Develop systems to encourage reporting of untoward events in the delivery of health care and offer immunity from litigation for such reports

However, there are major issues related to the internal workings of hospitals and medical staff governance over which physicians and health care professionals have sole control. A recent study, reported in the *New England Journal of Medicine,* indicated that as many as 36 percent of a large series of patients treated on the general medical service of a university hospital suffered some form of iatrogenic illness associated with their care.[2] Fully a quarter of these illnesses, affecting 9 percent of the patients treated, were life-threatening. In 1973, a government commission studying malpractice concluded that as many as one in three injuries occurring in hospitals is associated with physician negligence[3] (see figure 7.1).

If these statistics do, in fact, reflect the hospitalized population as a whole then providers may have experienced only a small proportion of the potentially valid malpractice cases to date. If there is a pool of potentially valid litigation that may be as large as two or three or even five percent of all

Figure 7.1. The Malpractice Pyramid

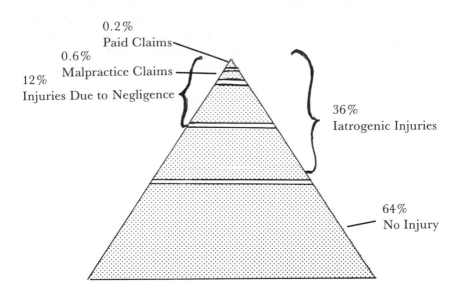

The percentages are estimated incidence of injuries, negligence-related injuries, claims, and compensated claims.

Sources of the data: National Assoication of Insurance Commissioners, 1980[1]; Steel, Gertman, and others, 1981[2]; and U.S. Department of Health, Education and Welfare, 1973.[3]

hospitalized patients, the approximately six-tenths of one percent currently involved in claims and the approximately two-tenths of one percent who receive compensation[4] are but a tiny fraction of the potential total.

It is becoming increasingly clear that, at least in part, the malpractice problem is associated with problems of quality of care, medical staff credentialing, and physician privilege delineation. Although there have been no national data collection efforts on medical professional liability since the publication of the final report of the National Association of Insurance Commissioners study in 1980,[4] these data and current experience suggest that 78 percent of all claims and 87 percent of total indemnity is associated with care provided in the hospital. Most of these claims arise from incidents that occur in the operating room, labor and delivery area, and the patient's room.

Comprehensive Risk Management

Currently, hospitals can employ two major approaches to minimize losses from medical malpractice claims: (1) reduce the risk of patient injury and (2) control claims by active intervention when injury occurs. Although both are important components of effective risk management, the second component, unfortunately, is often emphasized at the expense of the first. In many institutions, loss prevention has come to mean better patient relations and trying to develop a means for early intervention when an injury occurs and has the potential to lead to loss. If that is the sole focus of a hospital's risk management program, it misses the central issue: minimizing the risk of losses by reducing the likelihood of patient injury.

If, in fact, providers are to be successful in controlling medical liability losses, they must develop a more comprehensive program that strengthens quality control mechanisms and heightens clinicians' awareness of their role in avoiding malpractice liability. Eight specific steps can be taken to reduce the risk of patient injury.

1. Develop Improved Credentialing Procedures

Recent investigations have revealed that as many as 3,000 physicians may be practicing fraudulently in the United States, some with alleged diplomas purchased by mail. As a result, new scrutiny is being focused on the process of validating credentials to ensure that hospitals follow reasonable procedures in verifying the identity and training of applicants. There is substantial legal precedent holding that hospitals are responsible for making reasonable efforts not only to obtain pertinent information but to validate its accuracy as well. Institutions can no longer assume that information provided on an application is true. Rather, a systematic approach to validating information and obtaining adequate information in order to make a sound determination is becoming more critical.

Conversely, hospitals must also strive to ensure that staff privilege decisions are not based on the economic concerns of potential competitors. Because of the recent explosion in antitrust litigation, physicians who are potential competitors of an applicant should be careful to keep economic concerns from entering into the decision-making process.

Although the hospital's board of trustees remains ultimately responsible for the quality of patient care, its members are not in a position to judge quality directly and must, therefore, rely on the judgment of the medical staff regarding an applicant's qualifications. Systems of checks and balances, however, must be in place to maintain the accountability of the medical staff to the board for carefully evaluating quality of care considerations in making credentialing decisions. Key components of this evaluation include:

- *Validation of education.* Reviewers should validate the applicant's medical education, number of procedures performed and results obtained, residency training, and board certification status.
- *Liability experience.* Inquiries should be made of both the physician and his insurer regarding liability experience. Attempts should be made to validate the accuracy of the information supplied by the applicant with the insurer and with other institutions. Involvement in professional liability claims does not necessarily imply poor-quality medicine. Liability claims should, however, serve as a flag or indicator to alert the medical staff to the need for more careful evaluation of potential quality of care concerns.
- *Peer relationships.* Peer evaluations and the ability to work with others are important components of quality. However, care must be taken to ensure that consideration of such factors is specifically linked to the quality of services to be provided. In *Miller vs. Eisenhower Medical Center,*[5] the California Supreme Court held that unless a physician's personality problems posed a "clear and specific" threat to quality, those personality traits could *not* be used as the basis for denying medical staff membership.
- *Availability.* As good patient care requires that physicians be available and accessible within a reasonable period of time, availability is a valid criterion for staff membership. However, in defining this criterion, it is important to maintain some degree of flexibility. For instance, availability often cannot be measured by distance or time alone. In addition, reasonable availability of an obstetrician/gynecologist or anesthesiologist may differ substantially from that of a dermatologist or allergist.

Ultimately, the credentialing process is designed to ensure that applicants for privileges are capable of providing good patient care. If any of the evaluation components such as education, training, peer recommendations, or liability experience raise questions as to the quality of care that can be expected, it is both reasonable and necessary to extend the evaluation to an analysis of the process and outcomes of care provided by the applicant. The hospital may therefore request that the applicant produce copies of records for patients he has treated at other institutions.

Even if the questions about an applicant are based upon verbal information or on privileged information that cannot be obtained in writing, such review of patient records is appropriate. Hospitals have a great deal of latitude and discretion in their evaluation of an applicant's performance before admitting him or her to the staff, as the burden of proving competence is on the applicant. However, once the applicant is admitted to the staff or granted privileges, the burden shifts to the institution to prove that he or she is no longer competent, if termination of privileges becomes necessary. Consequently, one of the best places to control the quality of care in a hospital is at the "front end," through the credentialing process.

2. Improve Privilege Delineation

While the credentialing process examines an applicant's basic qualifications for admission to the staff or for the privilege to provide services, clinical privilege delineation serves as the "job description." The delineation of clinical privileges is a statement of the specific services that may be provided and of the types of patients who may be cared for by each medical staff member or individual granted privileges in the institution. The delineation tends to be different for each staff member, because seldom do two members of the staff have exactly the same experience, training, type of practice, and set of competencies.

In granting clinical privileges, common sense is important. Careful consideration should be given to the types of risks associated with the privileges that physicians are requesting. If they are requesting privileges for known high-risk procedures, then their training, experience, and results should be carefully examined. In addition, if the physicians are requesting privileges to perform uncommon procedures, such as jejunoileal bypasses, or are performing a high number of these procedures, the medical staff should raise questions regarding the appropriateness of the procedure. In one institution that had a large number of allegations of corporate liability pending, temporomandibular joint (TMJ) replacement was one of the leading surgical procedures performed. Common sense should indicate that it is unusual for TMJ replacement (or jejunoileal bypass) to rank as one of the most frequent procedures in any institution.

In granting clinical privileges, it is important to consider not only high-frequency or unusual procedures, but also low-frequency procedures as well. Skills in many areas of surgery are best maintained with high volume. According to the Stanford Institutional Differences Study,[6] mortality rates for a number of surgical procedures are directly related to volume. The higher the volume, the lower the mortality and the lower the morbidity rate. Conversely, lower volume tends to produce higher mortality rates.

If only six or seven esophagectomies are performed per year in a rural hospital and the mortality rate is 70 to 80 percent, the medical staff should question not only the surgeon's technical skill but whether or not the institution should even be performing that kind of high-risk procedure with such low frequency. Would it not be in the patients' best interests to refer them to a regional center for definitive care, where mortality statistics are more favorable?

Requests by members of the staff for privileges to perform newly developed procedures, such as chemonucleolysis, endoscopy, or laser procedures, should be carefully examined. As new procedures emerge, the institution and the medical staff should proactively set criteria for granting those privileges *in advance* of allowing the procedures to be performed. Thus, the delineation of privileges must change as medical technology changes, to ensure that the introduction of new procedures into the institution is firmly controlled by the medical staff.

Criteria for granting privileges to perform new procedures should state specifically the kind and extent of training that staff members must demonstrate. Too often, the medical staff learns that its members are already performing a procedure without any criteria in place for determining who should have the privilege. It is extremely difficult to define criteria retroactively, especially if it means removing a privilege which is already, de facto, in place. Accordingly, taking a proactive stance in delineating privileges for new procedures is a key to avoiding potential liability, divisions within the medical staff, and possible litigation regarding privileges.

3. Create Linkages between Quality Assurance and Privilege Renewal

The thrust of current quality assurance and medical staff standards of the Joint Commission on Accreditation of Hospitals (JCAH) is to establish firmer linkages between the review of quality and appropriateness of care by the medical staff and the renewal of clinical privileges. The purpose of a hospital quality assurance program is also to ensure that clinicians are competent and provide good care. Competence and judgment are always referenced in the medical staff bylaws as criteria for granting and renewing privileges.

The competence and clinical judgment of each practitioner should be demonstrated through the results of quality review activities, such as mortality review, antibiotic review, blood and tissue review, generic screening, incident report data, and liability claims data. These sources of information are available at any hospital and should be used to evaluate the competence and judgment of not only each member of the medical staff, but other individuals providing services. Renewal of clinical privileges should be based primarily on evaluation of this information.

To accomplish this objective, a "peer review file" should be established for each clinician with privileges. Although the information to be contained in this file is currently available in diverse locations throughout the institution, it should be collected into a single file for review as part of the privilege renewal process.

Physicians are very sensitive about the confidentiality of such data, however. Care must be exercised to assure that these files are kept in a locked file cabinet, and access to them should be very strictly controlled. A log should be kept, and anyone in a position of responsibility for medical staff governance who wishes to view a particular practitioner's file should sign the file out, state the reason for review, and return it to the locked cabinet promptly. That person should also be required to sign a confidentiality statement. Under no circumstances should the files be removed from the departmental or medical staff office. All individuals on the medical staff who have access to these files must respect the sensitive nature of information contained in them. At the same time, they must recognize the medical staff's responsibility to engage in a careful and systematic review of each physician's performance, as part of the privilege renewal process.

4. Increase Understanding of the Risks of Hospitalization

A growing body of literature now recognizes that as medicine has progressed and technologic sophistication has grown, so, too, have the risks. As noted earlier, a 1981 *New England Journal of Medicine* article reported that 36 percent of all patients hospitalized on the general medical service of a large university hospital incurred some type of iatrogenic illness that prolonged their stay.[2] Twenty-five percent of those illnesses were life-threatening.

Medical staffs must be made more aware of such statistics and of the kinds of clinical situations that carry high risk of patient injury and, therefore, high risk for potential litigation. Physicians are often lulled into a false sense of complacency by seeing the routine so frequently that they miss the unusual case that may represent a potential catastrophe.

A series of educational programs on the relationships between quality of care and the risk of malpractice litigation can go a long way toward alerting practitioners to high-risk areas and changing behavior in the care of these cases. Rather than a single 45-minute presentation, it is much more effective to provide smaller "doses" over a longer period of time and to focus not only on knowledge but also on attitudes.

In fostering positive attitudes toward loss prevention and quality improvement, positive reinforcement is much more effective than negative reinforcement. Accordingly, the educational series should emphasize the positive rewards to be attained by improving the quality of care, rather than the negative or punitive aspects of malpractice or other disciplinary mechanisms. In addition, medical staffs should consider various positive measures they can use to gain compliance with their own bylaws. For example, it may be much more effective to send letters to physicians congratulating them on the completeness and accuracy of their records than to notify them only when records are incomplete or delinquent. If the medical staff governance structure provides positive reinforcement for positive behavior, rather than only reprimands for negative behavior, physicians' long-term response to quality improvement efforts is likely to be more noticeable.

5. Enforce Medical Staff Rules and Regulations

Medical staff bylaws exist not only because they are required by the JCAH, but also because they are reasonable rules for operating an organized medical staff in a hospital setting. When the hospital, or its staff, fails to enforce its own bylaws, rules, regulations, or policies, it exposes the institution to potential liability and undermines the whole medical staff governance process. If bylaws are not applied equally to everyone, the medical staff's ability to govern itself may be substantially weakened. More simply stated, why should one physician follow the rules when other physicians are allowed to ignore them?

Recently, allegations have been brought against hospitals in malpractice claims charging that patients were injured because of the hospitals' failure to enforce their medical staff bylaws. A Florida hospital, for example, had enacted a policy requiring malpractice insurance of all physicians on the staff. A registered letter was sent to every physician informing him or her of this requirement. Subsequently, follow-up letters were sent to several physicians who had not produced the required certificate of insurance.

A staff orthopedic surgeon received yet a third letter, stating that, unless he submitted his certificate of insurance by a certain date, his privileges would be revoked. Soon after that date, the surgeon admitted a patient who had fallen, sustained a neck injury, and was experiencing paresthesia in her left arm. After conservative treatment with traction for four or five days, the physician performed a laminagram in which he saw a filling defect that led to an anterior cervical fusion. Postoperatively, the patient developed the Brown-Sequard syndrome and lost not only motor and sensory functions in her left side but also some bowel and bladder function.

During the subsequent litigation, it was discovered that the physician was uninsured and was about to file for bankruptcy. The plaintiff's attorneys brought an action against the hospital, alleging that it not only failed to enforce the insurance requirement, but also failed to enforce requirements for attendance at medical staff meetings, suspension for delinquent records, completion of a history and physical prior to surgery, and other provisions of the medical staff bylaws. The chief of this physician's department had never seen him operate, had not reviewed any of his records, and had no knowledge whatsoever of his competence or performance, yet had signed his renewal application for each of the last three biennial reappointments. When asked under oath why he had failed to evaluate the surgeon's competency, the chief of orthopedics said, "Because it's not nice and it's none of my business."[7]

Circumstances like this create the impression of a facility that does not enforce its own rules. Institutions like the Florida hospital are very vulnerable to allegations of negligence in patient injury cases and, accordingly, to liability.

6. Appoint Strong Department Chairmen

The role of clinical department chairmen is critical in preventing medical malpractice losses in hospitals. They have principal responsibility for enforcing medical staff bylaws, rules, and regulations, and for maintaining quality of care within their departments. Yet many chairmen are elected on the basis of popularity, rather than on their preparation for the duties and responsibilities of the position. Most chairmen have not been trained for their legal responsibilities, or in methods for carrying them out.

If hospitals are to achieve effective medical staff governance, they must recognize the key role of clinical department chairmen and ensure that they receive adequate training and education. Training in such areas as the legal responsibilities of department chairmen, methods for conducting effective meetings, techniques for uncovering and resolving conflict situations involving peers, and basic management methods are keys to successful medical staff governance. In addition, hospitals should recognize the substantial time commitment involved in being effective department chairmen and consider the issue of compensation.

7. Support the Actions of Department Chairmen

As important as strong department chairmen are to preventing malpractice losses, they cannot perform their duties unaided. Hospital procedures must be in place to document quality-of-care problems in the making. When chairmen prepare to take disciplinary action based on that documentation, they need to be assured of board and administration support.

The legal consequences of failing to act on known quality-of-care problems are generally more severe than are the consequences of reasonable, rational action taken on the basis of sound documentation. Unfortunately, however, hospitals often do not have the documentation necessary to take proper action.[8] If hospitals begin to create the linkages between quality assurance and credentialing discussed earlier, the documentation necessary for effective disciplinary action will be more readily available.

Once documentation procedures are established, it is critical that the institution support actions taken by department chairmen to enforce bylaws,

rules, and regulations, or to remedy quality-of-care deficiencies. No department chairman will long withstand the pressure that can be brought by
peers, if he or she is not supported by colleagues in the medical staff
governance structure, by the administration, and by the board of trustees.
The clinical department chairman must be assured that he or she can rely
upon the support of the board when it becomes necessary to take action to
enforce hospital policies and procedures or to take disciplinary actions
against a colleague.

In addition, the trustees must ascertain that all department chairmen
are taking their roles and responsibilities seriously. No chairman can continue to enforce department policies in the absence of strict enforcement in
other departments. Accordingly, the trustees may be faced with the necessity of removing an ineffective department chairman in order to support the
actions of stronger chairmen.

8. Improve Accountability between Medical Staff and Trustees

Historically, trustees have been reluctant to exercise their quality-of-care
responsibility, because they felt that this duty could be delegated to the
medical staff. Although many trustees do not have specific medical knowledge about quality-of-care issues, they do need to satisfy themselves that the
quality assurance mechanisms instituted by management and the medical
staff are adequate to control quality of care. Trustees must receive information on how these mechanisms are working to assure good professional
performance, low risk of patient injury, and effective use of hospital resources.[9]

The hospital board has four major objectives in its quality control
mission:

- To ensure that credentials and privileges are granted and renewed
  based on demonstrated competence and sound clinical performance
- To ensure that the hospital quality assurance program is effective
  in identifying, assessing, and resolving patient care problems
- To monitor institutional liability experience and take actions as
  required to reduce exposure to loss
- To ensure that employees are retained and promoted on the basis
  of competent performance[9]

Conclusion

Although the problem of medical malpractice is a complex one, involving
social, legal, and quality of care issues, effective actions by the hospital
medical staff can have a major impact on reducing the frequency of patient
injuries and strengthening the legal position of the hospital as a defendant.

By taking the eight steps discussed earlier for improving medical staff performance, hospitals should substantially lessen their malpractice liability exposure.

References

1. American Medical Association, Special Task Force on Professional Liability and Insurance. *Professional Liability in the 80s, Reports 1 and 2.* Chicago: AMA, 1984.
2. Steel, K., Gertman, P. M., and others. Iatrogenic illness on a general medical service at a university hospital. *New England Journal of Medicine.* 1981, Mar. 12. 304(11):638-642.
3. U.S. Department of Health, Education and Welfare. *Report of the Secretary's Commission on Medical Malpractice.* Washington, DC: U. S. Government Printing Office, 1973.
4. National Association of Insurance Commissioners. *Malpractice Claims: Final Compilation.* Brookfield, WI: NAIC, 1980.
5. Curran, W. J. Medical-staff privileges in private hospitals: Can modern hospitals exclude uncooperative applicants? *New England Journal of Medicine.* 1981 Mar. 5. 304(10):589-591.
6. Luft, H. S., Bunker, J. P., and Enthoven, A. C. Should operations be regionalized? The empirical relationship between surgical volume and mortality. *New England Journal of Medicine.* 1979 Dec. 20. 301(25):1364-1369.
7. *McWhirter vs. Deghan et al.,* Jacksonville, FL. Case settled prior to trial.
8. Jessee, W. F., and Brenner, L. H. Approaches to improving health care: dealing with the ''problem physician.'' *Quality Review Bulletin.* 1982. 8(1):11-14.
9. Jessee, W. F. *Quality of Care Issues for the Hospital Trustee.* Chicago: The Hospital Research and Educational Trust, 1984.

Chapter 8
Board Initiatives to Minimize the Risk of Hospital Liability

James J. Hughes, Jr.

There is an increasing move to impose responsibility on hospitals for ensuring the safety of medical treatment to patients. A 1973 survey, for example, estimated that between 75 and 80 percent of all malpractice claims arise in hospitals.[1] Moreover, hospitals are becoming de facto reinsurers of their medical staffs, as physicians find it harder to get malpractice insurance beyond a million dollars. In 1985 alone, some 26 insurance companies withdrew from the physician malpractice coverage business. Others saw their stock prices plummet.

Even though the basic goal of both hospitals and physicians is to provide high-quality health care in an efficient manner, mistakes will inevitably be made. In such situations, the question becomes, "Who will pay?" Eliminating direct hospital negligence, the patient's only recourse should be against the physician who committed the harmful act. However, where physicians are experiencing problems with coverage, plaintiffs' lawyers and the courts are increasingly looking to hospitals for responsibility.

Several legal theories have been developed to hold hospitals responsible for staff physicians' negligence. In addition to the traditional one of respondiate superior, the doctrines of corporate negligence, ostensible agency, and agency by estoppel are being involved. However, they are all basically the same in theory.

Corporate Negligence

The doctrine of corporate negligence imposes liability directly on hospitals, premised upon the hospital's failure to meet its duty to render high-quality medical care to its patients. In *Pedroza v. Bryant,* 677 P.2d 166 (1984), the Supreme Court of Washington based its ruling on this doctrine. The Court stated the issue as "(W)hether a hospital may be held liable under a theory of corporate negligence for its action in granting privileges to a nonemployee doctor who allegedly commits malpractice while in private practice off the hospital premises."

Mr. Hughes is an attorney with Bricker & Eckler, Columbus, OH.

Maria Pedroza was treated by Dr. Bryant during her 35th week of pregnancy. Although she exhibited classic symptoms of preeclampsia during her continued visits to his office, Dr. Bryant prescribed aspirin and bed rest. He did not refer Pedroza to another physician. She was later admitted, comatose, to the defendant hospital, where she died in surgery. Dr. Bryant was neither the admitting nor treating physician. According to his hospital privileges, Dr. Bryant would have been required in this case to have a consultation with a "class 1" physician.

Because there was no assertion that the hospital was negligent in the performance of any of the in-hospital treatment of Pedroza, the hospital moved to be dismissed from the case. The trial court granted the motion on the basis that: (1) the theory of hospital corporate negligence is not recognized in Washington, and (2) even if it were, the theory does not extend to acts done outside the hospital.

The Supreme Court affirmed this decision on the second grounds, but in doing so it expressly adopted the theory of corporate negligence. After adopting the theory of corporate negligence, the Court found the facts of the case to be too remote to find the hospital liable. In adopting the theory, the Court stated:

> The doctrine of corporate negligence (the label most commonly used) reflects the public perception of the modern hospital as a multifaceted health care facility responsible for the quality of medical care and treatment rendered. The community hospital has evolved into a corporate institution, assuming the role of a comprehensive health care center ultimately responsible for arranging and coordinating total health care....The patient treated in such a facility receives care from a number of individuals of varying capacities and is not merely treated by a physician acting in isolation.

> Today, in response to demands of the public, the hospital is becoming a community health center. The purpose of the community hospital is to provide patient care of the highest possible quality. To implement this duty of providing competent medical care to the patients, it is the responsibility of the institution to create a workable system whereby the medical staff of the hospital continually reviews and evaluates the quality of care being rendered within the institution.

> . . .The role of the hospital vis-a-vis the community is changing rapidly. The hospital's role is no longer limited to the furnishing of physical facilities and equipment where a physician treats his private patients and practices his profession in his own individualized manner.

Corporate negligence was first applied to hospitals in the landmark Illinois case of *Darling v. Charleston Community Memorial Hospital,* 33 Ill. 2d 326, 211 N.E. 2d 253 (1965), cert. denied, 383 U.S. 946 (1966). In *Darling,* the plaintiff broke his leg playing college football. At the defendant hospital, he was placed in a cast by a private staff physician. The staff physician applied the cast too tightly and without padding, resulting in the loss of the leg. Nurses and other witnesses had observed "blood and other seepage," as well as the odor of decaying flesh—clear signs of complications. Nonetheless, neither the physician nor other medical personnel had administered further treatment. The hospital also failed to investigate or review the admitting physician's work and failed to require a consultation, in disregard of a hospital medical staff bylaw requiring consultation in "all major cases."

The Illinois Supreme Court stated that a hospital owed a duty to render high-quality care and treatment to its patients. The court found the defendant hospital liable, based in large part upon its failure to follow its own rules and regulations, as well as generally accepted professional standards. The court stated that:

> The standards for hospital accreditation, the state licensing regulations, and the defendant's bylaws demonstrate that the medical profession and other responsible authorities regard it as both desirable and feasible that a hospital assume certain responsibilities for the care of the patient.

Board Responsibility

In *Darling* and several cases following it, the courts reference a number of standards by which a hospital's duty of care will be judged, including those published by the Joint Commission on Accreditation of Hospitals (JCAH). The court in *Pedroza,* for example, pointed to JCAH standards as establishing board responsibility for ensuring that the medical staff is acting properly:

> Perhaps the most important of the new national standards voluntarily adopted by hospitals are those promulgated by the JCAH. The JCAH standards clearly establish the institution's governing board as ultimately responsible for the overall quality of patient care provided in the hospital. *The medical staff, in turn, is responsible to the governing board for the professional competence of all physicians and dentists who are members of the hospital's medical staff.*
>
> The standards place particular emphasis on the appointment/ reappointment process, delineation of clinical privileges, and periodic appraisals of each physician staff member. In addition, the hospital is required to institute reliable and valid measures

that continuously evaluate the quality of care rendered all patients. JCAH accreditation means that a hospital has sufficiently complied with standards aimed at providing a comprehensive ongoing system of review capable of identifying any incompetent members of the medical staff. The standards could be valuable as a measure against which the hospital's conduct is judged to determine if the institution is meeting its duty of care to patients.

While the JCAH's medical staff standard VI requires the medical staff to "assume the provision of high-quality patient care through the monitoring and evaluation of the quality and appropriateness of patient care,[2] its governing body standard I states that:

An organized governing body, or designated persons so functioning, is responsible for establishing policy, maintaining quality patient care, and providing for institutional management and planning. In fact, a recurring theory throughout the JCAH standards is board involvement and supervision of medical staff programs of quality assurance.

A hospital's own bylaws also define its duty of care, as shown in *Scott v. Brookdale Hospital Center* 400 NYS 2d 552 (1977). A patient was brought to the defendant hospital after suffering a severe and incapacitating headache. The patient was examined by an intern who diagnosed his condition as gastroenteritis and released him the same day. One month later, the patient was again rushed to the hospital after suddenly falling down unconscious. Six days later, the patient died from a hemorrhage as a result of an aneurysm.

The plaintiff presented expert medical testimony showing that the deceased had suffered a "leak," or bleeding from an aneurysm located at the base of the brain. The expert testified that had the decedent been admitted to the hospital when he was first treated by the intern and undergone proper tests, the condition would have been discovered.

The expert further contended that the mere fact that the decedent suffered from such a headache was in and of itself enough to warrant certain tests and consultations with a neurologist or neurosurgeon. The court found that the hospital's failure to follow its own rules requiring such consultations constituted a departure from medical standards and therefore judged the hospital negligent.

In *Poor Sisters of St. Francis Seraph of Perpetual Adoration, Inc. v. Catron*, 435 N.E. 2d 305 (Ind. 1982), both a nurse and inhalation therapist failed to inform the attending physician that an endotracheal tube was being left in a patient longer than the customary three- to four-day period. They also failed to report the physician's treatment of the plaintiff to their supervisors. Based on these deviations from procedure, the court found the hospital liable.

These court cases illustrate the theories that courts will use to hold hospitals liable. But often, the courts "need" to hold the hospital liable because the physician's insurance limits are too low or the physician settled early and the only defendant left is the hospital (as in the *Darling* case). Whether courts hand down rulings based on need or legal theory, hospitals are now doubly vulnerable. Their boards, in turn, must become more active in monitoring the medical staff. Monitoring of staff physicians and execution of a proper program of quality assurance are fundamental responsibilities of a hospital board. This is the primary thrust of the JCAH standards, and it is an obligation that the courts will specifically require in the 1980s.

Minimizing the Risk

There are several steps hospitals can take to minimize their liability risk. Nine of them are discussed below, followed by a discussion of lawsuits that ensued when a hospital failed to implement each step.

1. Implement a mechanism to screen patients requiring emergency medical treatment, for which hospital facilities are inadequate, and transfer such patients to facilities that are adequately equipped to treat their conditions.

When JCAH teams conduct hospital site visits, they are looking for evidence of, among other things, a set plan for assessing emergency patients. As specified in JCAH standard I for emergency services:

A well-defined plan for emergency care, based on community need and the capability of the hospital, shall be implemented by every hospital.[2]

The interpretation of that standard spells out clearly a hospital's duty:

The hospital must have some procedure whereby the ill or injured person can be assessed and, as indicated, either treated or referred to an appropriate facility. Patients shall be transferred in accordance with the community-based hospital emergency plan. A hospital providing emergency care shall be capable of instituting essential life-saving measures and implementing emergency procedures that will minimize further compromise of the condition of any infant, child or adult being transported.[2]

In *Carrosco v. Bankoff*, 33 Cal Rptr. 673 (1963), a hospital was found liable for retaining a patient with third-degree burns for 53 days, when it did not offer facilities for the open method of treating burns or skin grafting. The court found that a duty arose to transfer the patient to another institution when the hospital did not have the facilities reasonably necessary to treat his condition. The *Darling* case is also an example of hospital failure to transfer a patient to a facility where proper care could be given.

2. Draft hospital medical staff bylaws that outline in detail careful appointment and reappointment procedures, including thorough investigation of credentials and prior medical experience, periodic reviews of physicians' competence and medical reporting, and documentation of such investigation.

In *Johnson v. Misericordia Community Hospital,* 99 Wis. 2d 708, 301 N.W. 2d 156 (1981), the court held the defendant hospital liable for the malpractice of an incompetent surgeon whom it had appointed to the staff without investigation. The finding of negligence was based in part on the foreseeability that a hospital's failure to properly investigate and verify the accuracy of an applicant's statements about his training, experience, and qualifications presents an unreasonable risk of harm to its patients.

The court in *Pedroza* also stated that "hospitals are in a superior position to that of state licensing boards, professional organizations, and the Professional Standards Review Organizations Program to monitor and control physicians' medical performance" (*Pedroza* p. 169).

3. Ensure that medical staff committees responsible for the review of physicians' performance conduct thorough reviews of all matters, including malpractice claims involving staff physician competency that come to their attention.

In *Purcell v. Zimbelman,* 18 Ariz. App. 75, 500 P. 2d 335 (1972), Dr. Purcell was found negligent in his performance of abdominal surgery. Tucson General Hospital was also found liable on the theory that it knew or should have known that Dr. Purcell lacked the skill to perform the operation. Evidence that Dr. Purcell had been twice successfully sued for malpractice in the performance of the identical surgical procedure was presented.

The court rejected the hospital's defense of lack of knowledge, premised on the fact that the suits were presented to the department of surgery, which was comprised of independent staff physicians. The court reasoned that the hospital had assumed the duty of supervising the competence of its staff members and thus could be held responsible for the department's failure to ensure that action be taken against Dr. Purcell or to recommend to the board of trustees that action be taken.

Although the filing of a lawsuit does not prove anything, recurring suits against a physician should prompt a performance review. By the same token, the outcome of a case is not pertinent. What a jury decides is not a material consideration in determining a physician's competence. However, court actions should put the credentials committee on notice to conduct an independent evaluation.

4. Conduct an independent review on a regular basis of decisions made by the credentials committee and of physician performance reviews made by the medical staff.

In *Gonzales v. Nork,* No. 228566 (Sacramento Super. Nov., 1973) rev'd 60 Cal. App 3d 728, 132 Cal Rptr 717 (1976), Aff'd on other grounds 20 Cal. 3d 500, 143 Cal. Rptr 240, 573 P. 2d 458 (1978), the hospital was found liable for allowing a physician to perform a laminectomy despite his incompetence, which the court held should have been known by the hospital. Evidence proved that Dr. Nork had performed 50 incompetent and unnecessary operations on 38 patients, made fictitious entries in his medical reports, deceived patients in order to obtain surgical consent, and discouraged patients from consulting other physicians.

The court found the hospital liable for failing to supervise Dr. Nork's patient care, despite the hospital's contention that its standards of review met JCAH requirements. The court deemed the standards insufficient in that:

- They were predicated on the assumption that the doctor was reporting honestly and that the records were truthful and accurate. Such assumptions cannot be made, since the hospital has a duty to protect its patients against fraudulent doctors.
- The required clinical review was subjective according to the personal standards of the reviewer. The review in court showed that such a subjective review will not disclose known deficiencies.
- The review was random. Therefore, bad cases were picked up only by chance.
- The review was infrequent.
- The review was casual, uncritical, and sandwiched in between the doctors' other work.
- The review did not include a comparison of the doctors' progress records and the nurses' notes.
- No protocol, profile, or record was made of doctors' deficiencies so that there was no common fund of knowledge available to the hospital.

In essence, hospital boards must determine if medical staff committees are functioning effectively and not merely acting pro forma. There should be reports from the committees to the board, joint seminars, discussions at joint conference committee meetings, medical staff briefings to the board, and visits to committee meetings by board members.

5. Delete any language from hospital bylaws that "assures" or "guarantees" a certain level of patient treatment above the standard of non-negligence. Otherwise the hospital's bylaws may be used in malpractice cases as evidence of the standard of care applicable to the hospital.

Medical staff bylaws are routinely used in malpractice cases (*Pedroza* and *Johnson,* for example) as evidence of the standard of care to which physicians practicing at a particular hospital should be held. The normal standard of care is one of non-negligence. However, any language in the bylaws that "assures" or "guarantees" a higher level of treatment could arguably create expectations that the public is entitled to receive a higher level than that of non-negligence.

In *Pulvers v. Kaiser Foundation Health Plan,* 160 Cal Rptr. 392 (1979), the plaintiff claimed that the language contained in the plan's literature represented it as providing "high standards of medical service." The plan's physicians should therefore be held to a higher standard of care than that of non-negligence, the plaintiff argued. Although the California Court of Appeals rejected that argument, the fact that the language resulted in a lawsuit is reason enough for deleting similar superlative language from hospital bylaws.

6. Draft medical staff bylaws that limit a physician's clinical privileges to the procedures he can competently perform.

In *Corleto v. Shore Memorial Hospital,* 138 N.J. 302, 350 A. 2d 534 (1975), the plaintiff's daughter died following abdominal surgery. The court allowed the plaintiff to proceed against the hospital, explaining that a hospital could be liable for permitting a physician to perform an operation he was incompetent to undertake, because it had wrongfully placed an incompetent in a position where he could do harm.

To avoid potential liability, hospitals should therefore ensure that medical staff bylaws acknowledge physician differences in background, training, experience, and skill level in the granting of privileges. Rather than simply making an applicant "a member of the department of surgery with orthopedic privileges," the medical staff should specify which procedures the physician may undertake.

7. Continuously update the medical accuracy of all hospital policies and procedures enacted for the protection of patients.

In *Air Shields, Inc. v. Spears,* 590 S.W. 2d 574 (Tex App. 1979), the defendant hospital was found liable because it adhered to procedures and policies that were based on questionable medical accuracy. The case revolved around a premature baby who was placed in an incubator and administered oxygen of 32 to 40 percent, resulting in total blindness.

Evidence produced during the trial showed that hospital procedure permitted oxygen administration to newborns of up to 40 percent, when ordered by a doctor. But medical knowledge at the time considered the practice dangerous and that oxygen should not be routinely given to newborns. There was no evidence that other hospitals had policies similar to the defendant hospital's. In fact, two hospitals in the area had policies designed to avoid routine administration of oxygen. On the basis of this evidence, the court found that the hospital could be held liable for negligent formulation of medical rules and procedures.

In another case, *Tonsic v. Wagner,* 220 Pa. Super Ct. 468, 289 A. 2d 138 (1974), the Pennsylvania Supreme Court held that a hospital could be found liable for negligence in a case where it was contended that the establishment of guidelines for a surgical-instrument count could have prevented the plaintiff's injury.

8. Regularly monitor compliance with hospital bylaws, policies, and procedures.

As discussed in *Darling,* a hospital owes a nondelegable duty of care to its patients. A hospital's failure to render responsible patient care by monitoring and enforcing its own bylaws can easily lead to liability. The hospital's duty to monitor compliance applies not only to the medical staff but to all persons within the hospital community.

In *Pederson v. Dumouchel,* 72 Wash. 2d 73, 431 P. 2d 973 (1967), the court found the hospital negligent, as a matter of law, for permitting a dentist on its staff to operate on a patient under general anesthesia without a medical doctor present, in violation of its own rules.

To effectively monitor compliance, a hospital's board members can take turns sitting as observers on quality assurance (QA) committees. As a minimum, the minutes of QA committees should be presented to the board and an actual report of committee activities made at board meetings.

The growing number of allied health practitioners makes board involvement even more pertinent today. The board must determine their scope of privileges, their relationship to the medical staff, and the method of credentialing. Most of the rules that apply to the medical staff should be extended to allied health professionals as well.

9. Require all staff physicians to carry adequate malpractice insurance.

In events leading up to *Holmes v. Hoemako,* 117 Ariz 403, 573 P. 2d 477 (1977), a staff physician informed the hospital board that he had chosen not to renew his professional liability insurance policy. After an administrative hearing, the staff physician was suspended. In holding for the hospital, the court stated that it was not unreasonable or arbitrary for a hospital to establish rules requiring its staff physicians to carry professional liability insurance.

The physician without or with too little insurance is a threat to the hospital and other staff physicians. To ensure compliance with these rules, physicians should be asked to file a copy of their insurance policy with the hospital. A member of the administrative staff should also review those files regularly to make sure they contain up-to-date policies.

Conclusion

Hospitals are increasingly being found liable for malpractice that occurs to patients while they are within hospital walls. *Darling* and other cases have imposed on hospitals nondelegable duties to render high-quality medical care to patients. Only the board has the authority to require that the medical staff perform its role of quality assurance.

When hospitals are found liable in a court case, it is not usually because they failed to establish proper policies and procedures. The policies are usually in place, but they were not enforced. Typically, a plaintiff's attorney will use hospital rules and procedure to prove that they either were inadequate to protect his client or were not followed, resulting in harm to his client. Hospitals should, therefore, affirmatively defend against corporate liability by carefully drafting hospital bylaws and diligently adhering to them. The board, in turn, must demand adherence.

References

1. U.S. Department of Health, Education, and Welfare. *Report of the Secretary's Commission on Medical Malpractice.* Washington, DC: U.S. Government Printing Office, 1973.
2. Joint Commission on Accreditation of Hospitals. *Accreditation Manual for Hospitals.* 1985 ed. Chicago: JCAH, 1985.